# Yoga to Go

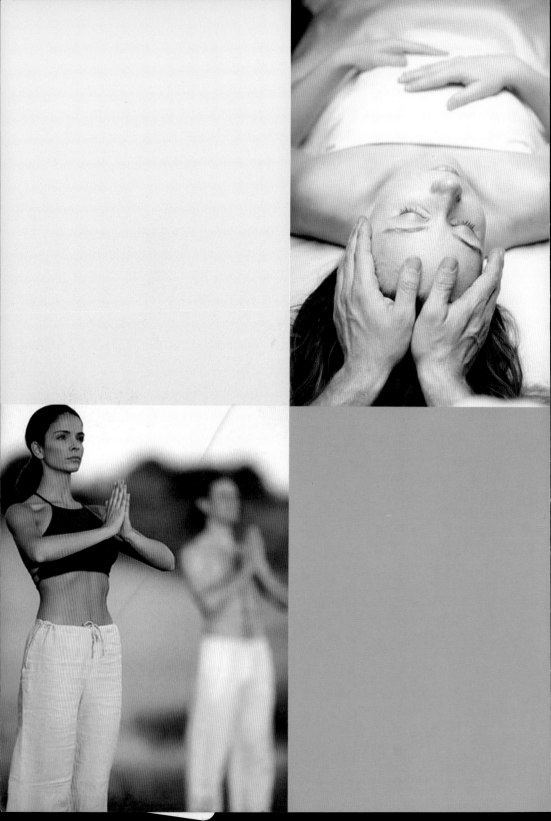

PAULA CARINO

# Yoga to Go

ILLUSTRATIONS BY
TRACEY WOOD

A take-it-with-you

guide for travelers

STERLING PUBLISHING CO., INC.
NEW YORK

Edited by Hazel Chan

Design by Kay Schuckhart/Blond on Pond

Photos for Chapters Two and Three, and page 224 by David Allee and Sarah Silver

**Library of Congress Cataloging-in-Publication Data**

Carino, Paula.

  Yoga to go / Paula Carino.

      p. cm.

  Includes index.

  ISBN 0-8069-8032-X

1. Yoga, Hatha. 2. Travel–Health aspects. 3. Mind and body. I. Title.

RA781.7 .C359 2004

613.7'046–dc22                                                         2003019013


10  9  8  7  6  5  4  3  2  1


Published by Sterling Publishing Co., Inc.

387 Park Avenue South, New York, NY 10016

© 2004 by Paula Carino

Distributed in Canada by Sterling Publishing

<sup>c</sup>/o Canadian Manda Group, One Atlantic Avenue, Suite 105

Toronto, Ontario, Canada M6K 3E7

Distributed in Great Britain by Chrysalis Books Group PLC

The Chrysalis Building, Bramley Road, London W1O 6SP, England

Distributed in Australia by Capricorn Link (Australia) Pty. Ltd.

P.O. Box 704, Windsor, NSW 2756, Australia

# DEDICATION

This book is dedicated to you, the reader.
Thank you for letting me serve you.

# ACKNOWLEDGMENTS

I'd like to thank the following for their support
and encouragement:
My parents, Robert Carino and the late Helene Carino.
My husband, David Wechsler, my parents-in-law, Bruce and Sandy
Wechsler, and Melody Wechsler.
Swami Satchidananda and the yogis and yoginis at Satchidananda
Ashram (Yogaville) and Integral Yoga of New York.
My students.
The luminous souls who agreed to be interviewed for this book.
Zelina Blagden, for embodying yoga.
My editors at Sterling, Danielle Truscott and Hazel Chan.
David Allee and Sarah Silver, for a fun and effortless photo shoot.
My two upward-facing dogs, Brighton and Mercy.

# Contents

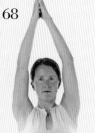

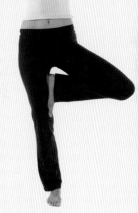

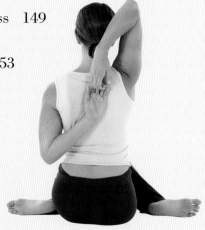

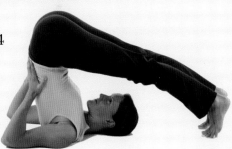

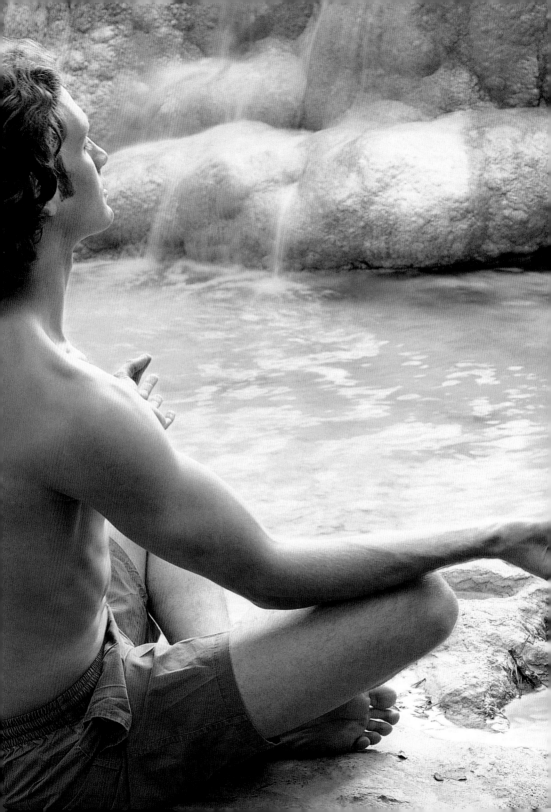

# The Journey

At no time are we ever in such complete possession of a journey, down to its last nook and cranny, as when we are busy with preparations for it. After that, there remains only the journey itself, which is nothing but the process through which we lose our ownership of it.

—Yukio Mishima (*Confessions of a Mask,* New Directions Publishing Corporation)

This book is not about yoga vacations, or about how to sign up for exotic (and expensive) Ashtanga retreats in Anguilla, or about getting away from your life in order to do yoga. This book is a guide for taking the ancient practices of hatha yoga with you into the many planned and unplanned adventures of your travel. Whether your trip is for business or pleasure, the disruption of your daily routine can become stressful. Yoga, one of the oldest forms of stress-management known to civilization, can help keep you centered and energized by bringing together the mind, body, and spirit through a set of physical exercises known as postures (or to use the Sanskrit term, *asanas*).

The *asanas* and breathing exercises (*pranayama*) in this book are easy to learn and do not require complicated props or lots of advanced training. If you are a complete novice to yoga, it might be worthwhile to take a few yoga classes before you travel. This way, you can experience how the postures should look and feel under the guidance of a good yoga teacher. You can also use this opportunity to ask the yoga teacher any questions you might have about modifying the postures to your own body type or limitations.

## HOW TO USE THIS BOOK

Chapter One covers some of yoga's basic principles, which will help keep you in a peaceful frame of mind when you travel. The next two chapters deal with the physical practices of yoga. There are thousands of known *asanas* in yoga. My intention is to boil them down into a basic series of therapeutic postures that you can take with you on your trip and keep with you for the rest of your life. Let the postures described in Chapter Two serve as ingredients and the routines outlined in Chapter Three the recipes for a healthy and balanced yoga program on the road. Chapter Four discusses some ways to make healthy food choices as you travel as well as what foods can help you if you experience certain ailments. Chapter Five covers meditation and includes some guided meditations to accompany you on your trip.

The rewards of a steady yoga practice are the tools that a person needs most in his or her travels: patience (in the face of lost luggage and long lines), good will toward strangers (even the rude airport clerk who tells you your reservation is missing), a trust in the flow of life (when the details of your trip spin out of control), and glowing physical health (to stave off the effects of dehydration, fast food, and jet lag). Most important, as you reap the benefits of yoga for your outward journey, you will find that it also sets you on an inward journey of self-discovery. Whichever path you take, enjoy your trip!

# CHAPTER ONE

# Thoughts for Traveling

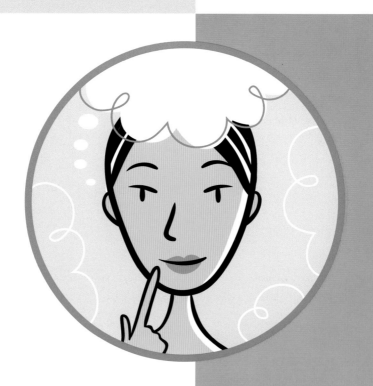

The true task of spiritual life

is not found in faraway places

or unusual states of consciousness.

It is here in the present.

It asks of us a welcoming spirit

to greet all that life presents to us

with a wise, respectful, and kindly heart.

—Jack Kornfield (*After the Ecstasy, the Laundry: How the Heart Grows Wise on the Spiritual Path*, Bantam Books)

## YOGA'S EIGHT LIMBS

The word "yoga" comes from the Sanskrit word *yuj*, which means to bind and is often translated as "union." Yoga is a practice of achieving union with your true nature by purifying your body and mind. It's not enough to just *know* that your true nature is divine. You need practices to anchor yourself to this deeper reality.

Thousands of years ago, the Indian sage Patanjali gathered the basic doctrines of yoga into 195 aphorisms, which were memorized and handed down orally by yogis for generations. These sayings eventually became known as the *Yoga Sutras*, which describe yoga's aims, methods, and benefits. In the *Sutras*, Patanjali mentions yoga's eight limbs, or practices. To purify the body and mind, end suffering, and achieve union with the divine, these eight limbs are to be observed faithfully:

1. The *Yamas* (behavior toward others)
2. The *Niyamas* (behavior toward ourselves)
3. *Asana* (postures)
4. *Pranayama* (breathing exercises)
5. *Pratyahara* (sense withdrawal)
6. *Dharana* (concentration/contemplation)
7. *Dhyana* (meditation)
8. *Samadhi* (bliss)

These limbs progress from outward concerns to increasingly more inward concerns. The first two limbs, the *yamas* and *niyamas*, deal with ethical and psychological issues. There are five *yamas* (*ahimsa, satya, asteya, brahmacharya,* and *aparigraha*) and five *niyamas* (*saucha, santosa, tapas, svadhyaya,* and *isvara pranidhana*). Together they lay a wonderful groundwork for the traveling yogi. Let's look at each one as it relates to travel.

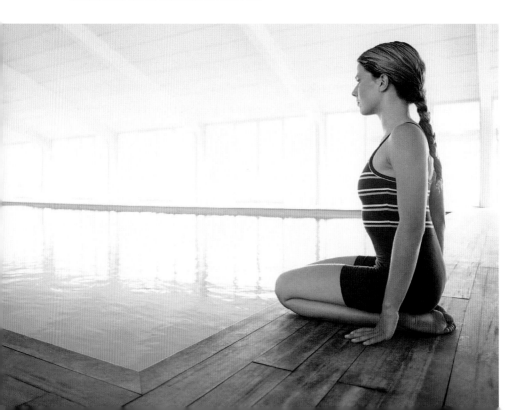

# THE *YAMAS*: THE CONSCIOUS TRAVELER

The first *yama* is *ahimsa*, or nonharming. Stated positively, *ahimsa* is helpfulness and compassion toward yourself and others. In a sense, it is the ethic that underlies all the other precepts in yoga's eight-limbed tree. Traveling presents us with many opportunities to demonstrate graciousness and nonharming.

If you have ever had to deal with flight delays or being stuck in a traffic jam, you can understand how quickly traveling puts you in a "wanting" state of mind. Your focus becomes so solely fixed upon achieving your aim and you feel so helpless in the situation that any additional inconvenience—the rude airport personnel or the car that cut in front of you—can feel many times worse than if you encountered it under ordinary circumstances.

The observance of *ahimsa* can dissolve that wanting feeling. Instead of feeling as though it is you against the world, you can approach each travel scenario from a standpoint of "How can I help? How can I bring peace to this situation?"

For example, let's say that you are boarding a plane and someone is blocking the aisle trying to get his luggage in the overhead compartment. Your first response may be to feel irritated or to complain inwardly, maybe even outwardly, about the person's selfishness or clumsiness. But a second response, in the spirit of *ahimsa*, can be to take a deep breath and ask the person if he needs a hand. The soothing effect of helping, or even just offering and reaching out in a friendly way, can erase the initial annoyance.

When visiting a foreign culture, *ahimsa* may take the form of honoring local customs and practices: respecting dress codes and demonstrating concern toward the environment, people, and animals that inhabit a place.

*Ahimsa* also means caring for yourself. When tension runs high, *ahimsa* can mean taking a moment to breathe deeply, close your eyes, and check in to see how you're feeling. You can summon the wisdom of your body and ask, "What do you need right now at this moment?" With awareness and concern for yourself, you can stay centered enough to be a helpful presence to others.

The second *yama* is *satya*, or truthfulness. Keeping secrets or covering up dishonesty creates stress in the body and mind. Being in an unfamiliar place can give you many chances to misrepresent the truth, because you might feel that the truth won't catch up with you. You will never see these people again. In the yogic philosophy, it's believed that the more you tell the truth, the more the outside world begins to reflect your truth. In other words, when you have a pure conscience, your thoughts and intentions carry more creative power.

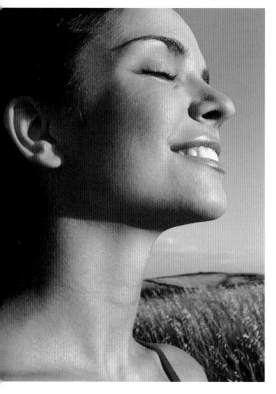

The third *yama* is *asteya*, or non-stealing and respect for the belongings of others. According to the wisdom of yoga, to steal is to go against your higher Self, which provides you with everything you need. Of course, most people would never consciously steal or shoplift, but while traveling, how many times does one carelessly take or disrespect the property of others? For example, taking hotel towels may seem like standard practice, but those thefts do add up. In some places (for instance, Mexico), the hotel cleaning staff is held responsible for bed clothes and towels, so stolen linens may be paid for out of the maid's salary.

Haggling for goods and services until a price is too low for the seller to make a profit can be seen as another form of stealing. Taking pictures without asking permission or picking flowers from someone else's property can be a form of theft too. By making an effort not to steal on any level, you strengthen your bond with the forces that provide for you (providence). You can practice both *asteya* and *ahimsa* by simply making a commitment to spend your money on local food, entertainment, and lodging so that the earnings stay in the community.

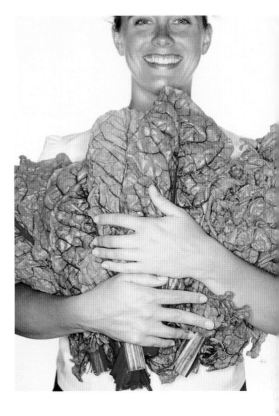

*Brahmacharya* is the fourth *yama*. For monks, *brahmacharya* is celibacy, or channeling sexual energies toward higher purposes. For the rest of the world, *brahmacharya* translates as moderation and continence—controlling sensual desires for your own well-being. In either context, *brahmacharya* preserves your limited economy of energy.

When you go on vacation, your impulse to overindulge in food, drink, and late nights may lead you to the point where you need a vacation after your vacation, which seems self-defeating. For the practicing yogi, a vacation can be an opportunity to take a break from your daily routine and explore with a steady mind the marvels of another place. You can also use this time as a chance to self reflect or to begin new routines or diets that would be difficult to start at home. When you travel on business, it's even more important to practice restraint, or *brahmacharya*, in order to focus your energies toward the work you need to do.

The fifth *yama* is *aparigraha*, which means noncovetousness or nonhoarding. On a basic level, *aparigraha* keeps your load light. When traveling, your impulse may be to take some part of your trip home with you, whether it is through buying a souvenir or taking a picture. Of course these are normal things that everybody does on vacation, but it may be worthwhile to study the intentions behind the actions (see *svadhyaya*, page 23). Are you taking home souvenirs to give to others and share the beauty of your experience with them, or are you holding on to the experience of your trip because you are afraid of letting this happy moment go? Will you be able to integrate all the things you've gathered on your trip into your life back home, or will they simply clutter up your living space and block your energies?

There is no absolute right or wrong answer, but these questions may provide insight into your thoughts and behavior.

## THE *NIYAMAS*: THE BALANCED TRAVELER

The next limb of the yoga tree is composed of the *niyamas*. These are observances that purify you and open you up to your true blissful nature.

The first *niyama* is *saucha*, or purity. Physical purity strengthens both the body and mind, freeing you to enjoy your travels. Purity includes maintaining good personal hygiene even when it may be a challenge. (This is where a good travel toothbrush and hand sanitizer come in.) It also means eating healthy, fresh foods and drinking clean water whenever possible (see Chapter Four), and keeping your personal spaces (car, airplane seat, workstation, hotel room) tidy and

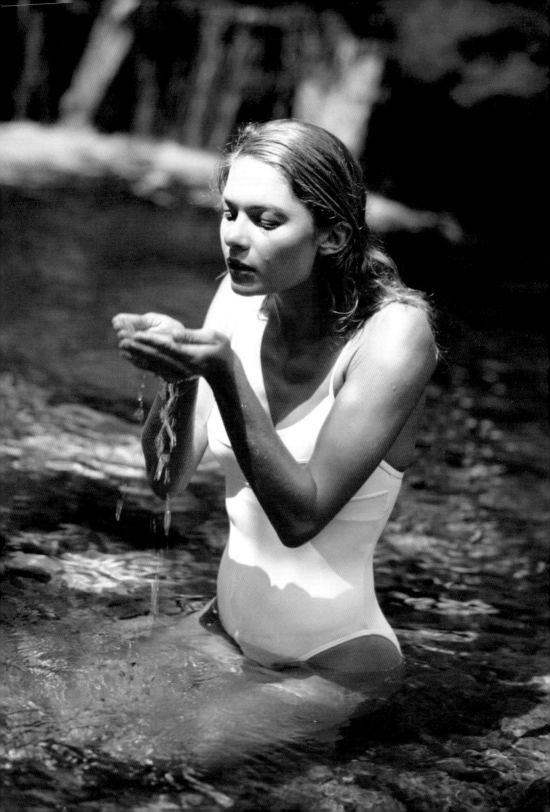

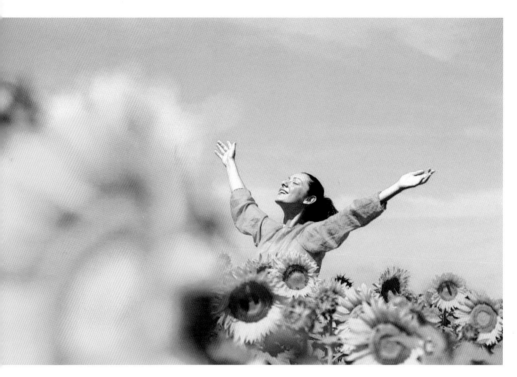

ordered, not just for your own peace of mind, but with compassion for the next person who inhabits the space. When you faithfully practice purity, you are able to delight in the more subtle pleasures of your travels, such as the sun on your skin and the new-car smell inside a rental car.

The second *niyama* is *santosa*, or contentment. Linked strongly with *aparigraha*, *santosa* is the habit of simply reveling in the present condition of your life without grasping for things beyond your reach. *Santosa* sings through you when you are satisfied with who you are, what you have, and what you do. An attitude of *santosa* transforms most travel experiences into joyous ones, because you have resolved to be content in the moment, whether you're sitting on a lovely beach or a not-so-lovely bench in a bus depot. For the traveler practicing *santosa*, sitting on a bench can be transformed into an impromptu meditation session (see Chapter Five), a fun stretch of people watching, a chance for writing in your journal, or even a heartfelt conversation with the stranger next to you. By observing *santosa*, you commit to spotting the good in your life rather than chasing after what you perceive to be someone else's good fortune.

The next three *niyamas* are closely related, and are often discussed as a triumvirate called the *kriyas*, or sacred actions. They are *tapas* (discipline), *svadhyaya* (self-study), and *isvara pranidhana* (honoring a higher power).

Though *tapas* translates from the Sanskrit as "heat," the word embraces other meanings, from "austerity" to "tolerance" to "discipline." Imagine a great refining fire burning inside of you. It may be painful at first, but the fire is making you shine brighter and purer. That is *tapas*, the "heat" of discipline. As a traveler, you need discipline to stick with your yoga practice when it's more convenient to skip it, and you need patience and fortitude when travel mishaps challenge even your most enthusiastic *santosa*.

*Tapas* asks you to bear annoyances, pain, and suffering with quiet dignity. In your travels, you may visit a culture where there is grinding poverty or overt racism or sexism. You may be asked to fly halfway around the globe for a half-hour business meeting. You may encounter hostility or violence on foreign soil. None of these experiences need to be denied or glossed over, but *tapas* asks you to allow the inevitable suffering of life to transform you into a better, more compassionate and alive person. Bearing the slings and arrows of life encourages a suppleness of character and ability to look at the world unflinchingly.

*Svadhyaya* follows closely on the heels of *tapas*. It means "self-study" both in the sense of studying scriptures independently and studying yourself with detachment and respect. This observance

Travel gives us the opportunity to bring the spirit of yoga to all persons and situations that we may encounter. Being present, aware, and receptive to what is going on is not just for our hatha classes. Truly practicing yoga is a 24/7 commitment. Respecting others, even if our relationship to them is fleeting—that is our real practice.

—Mara Carrico, yoga teacher, author of *Yoga Journal's Yoga Basics: The Essential Beginner's Guide to Yoga for a Lifetime of Health and Fitness* (Henry Holt & Company, Inc.), choreographer of *Jane Fonda's Yoga Exercise Workout* video

ensures that yoga does not become something that you follow blindly, but rather a living laboratory of observation. Yoga is experiential. Nothing about it is taken on authority or faith. Instead, you constantly witness your own response to the postures, to the *yamas* and *niyamas*, and decide for yourself if they are working to promote peace and healing within you. The more you dispassionately observe your behavior, the better position you are in to change the behaviors that don't work and keep the ones that do. And the closer you follow your behavior, the more subtle your awareness becomes.

Travel allows you to examine your behavior and attitudes away from the comfortable routines and relationships that fortify your identity at home. Two of the best travel companions are a journal for writing impressions, thoughts, and visions, and inspiring literature or the sacred texts of your religion. When faced with a five-hour flight or train ride, you can resist the urge to zone out in front of a magazine or mystery novel and pick up some uplifting literature or your journal. It helps keep your mind focused on your highest values, making it easier to remember your true identity.

*Isvara pranidhana* means actively honoring the spiritual dimension of life—the higher power that resides inside you and all around you. Surrendering is sometimes scary because you don't want to be defeated or humiliated, but *isvara pranidhana* asks you to surrender to the best parts of yourself: the loving, rational, guiding, self-sustaining impulses that can get blocked by your ego's selfish and destructive demands. *Isvara* can manifest as an unabashed, fluid sense of wonder at the benevolent forces flowing through, around, under, and above you.

Imagine that there is a shimmering light emanating from all living things—a light of pure love. When you can "see" that light behind every face you meet on your journey and respond with compassion, then you are practicing *isvara pranidhana*. The more you allow that light to shine, the more it appears on your path, lighting the way ahead for a smoother ride.

## THE REST OF THE LIMBS: THE MEDITATIVE TRAVELER

The next two limbs of the yogic tree, *asanas* (postures) and *pranayama* (breathing exercises) are what almost everyone identifies as "yoga." We'll be exploring those limbs in depth in Chapters Two and Three.

The fifth limb, *pratyahara*, is the act of retracting the senses away from their respective objects, or temporarily withdrawing from the senses in order to attain a deep state of relaxation, and contemplating a deeper, more subtle level of being. This all sounds pretty esoteric, but it is actually quite easy to start down the road to *pratyahara* by practicing a deep relaxation technique called Yogic Sleep, or *Yoga Nidra* (see pages 100–104).

Holding yoga poses, performing breathing exercises, and relaxing deeply will refresh and strengthen the physical body in measurable ways, but in the complete eight-limbed system, these practices are meant to prepare the body and mind for the next two limbs: *dharana* (concentration) and *dhyana* (meditation).

Concentration is an act of the will: focusing awareness on an object, such as a mantra (a sound or word), your breath, or a candle flame, until the many images, memories, and sounds inside your mind quiet down and become replaced with more and more subtle perceptions. With enough repetition and commitment in concentration, you may get to a point where your mind flows effortlessly toward complete stillness. From that stillness, you can perceive who you

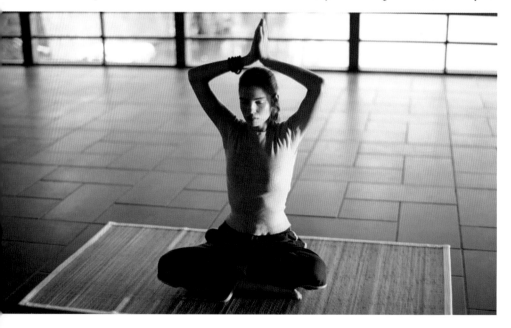

Being on the road can be very taxing for the body and disturbing for the mind. It is essential to have an action plan to stay calm and balanced. Bringing along some personal items for your room, like a picture, music, candles, incense, bath salts, or whatever helps you stay calm. I try and take each challenge with calm. If I have to stay in an airport for awhile, I just take advantage of the time. Some of my best work occurs in some of the worst circumstances!

—Darrin Zeer, world traveler and author of *Office Yoga: Simple Stretches for Busy People* (Chronicle Books)

really are. You become pure awareness. This effortless awakening of perception and knowledge is called meditation, or *dhyana* (see Chapter Five).

The last limb, *samadhi*, is the result of all your yogic exploration. It can be described as a permanent state of meditation, a locked-in sense of oneness with the radiant source of the universe. It is not something that you can willfully experience, but you practice with the intention that someday, in this lifetime or the next, you will arrive at this enlightened destination.

But let's not worry about all that right now. You have a trip to take.

# CHAPTER TWO

# The Postures

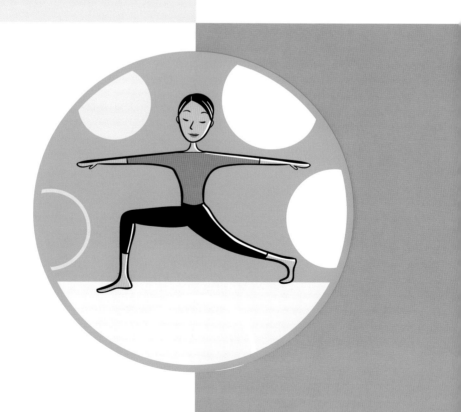

When your yoga becomes part

of you, it "does you" as much as you do it.

—Ganga White

Practicing yoga postures, or *asanas*, is a perfect example of "traveling without arriving." There's no point at which you can accurately say, "I've come to the end of the line—there's no more to explore." There is always more to explore because the postures aren't fixed and your body and mind are always evolving. You come to *asana* practice to strengthen and relax your body, but you do so with an attitude of observation, investigating the interaction of the postures with your body and mind on any given day. You notice connections, such as: "Today I'm struggling to hold Downward Facing Dog. Yesterday it was effortless. What's going on here?"

The value of your practice is in the quality of your awareness. It doesn't depend on how "well" you hold the postures, or how you compare to other people or an idea of perfection. What matters is staying present with all the sensations that the posture induces and keeping your breath steady.

Good results come from just trying, even if you don't look like a picture from a yoga book. Experiment with unfurling your body into the postures. Take your time instead of zipping right into them and holding them rigidly. Allow the postures to breathe through you.

For other practical considerations before you begin your practice, see "How to Start and End a Session," pages 110–112.

## SAFETY GUIDELINES

The postures presented in this book are suitable for beginners and people at most ability levels. However, you know your own body better than anyone. If you have an injury, chronic illness, or haven't exercised in a long time (or ever), please consult a health professional before trying hatha yoga. A physician or experienced yoga teacher may be able to prescribe modified postures to mesh with your unique limitations and abilities. Those limitations and abilities often change daily, especially under travel conditions. Let your body "tell" you how far it wants to go on any given day. Do not force or strain.

If you haven't exercised in a while, the movements and stretching of the postures may awaken new sensations in your body. Usually those sensations are wonderful, but occasionally they may be uncomfortable—either physically or emotionally. Do your best to distinguish between the ache of awakening a tight muscle and the pain of overdoing it. Acute or excruciating pain is never a good sign. Stop immediately if you experience a sharp pain during a stretch.

Each of the poses in this book has a modification section to help you adjust the pose to your body's needs. Refer to them before beginning a pose.

## MENSTRUATION

Various hatha yoga traditions differ in their attitudes toward menstruation: some believe that menstruating women should only practice breathing exercises (*pranayama*) and meditation, and omit doing postures, for the duration of their period; others believe that menstruation should not deter a woman from her usual practice. Most take the middle road, suggesting that you stay extra attentive to your body's promptings and be willing to forgo postures that make you uncomfortable.

Many schools discourage inversions, such as Shoulder Stand (*Sarvangasana*; see pages 76–78), for menstruating women, although it has not been scientifically proven that being upside down disrupts the menstrual flow. Some women report discomfort in inverted postures and postures that put pressure on the abdomen, such as The Bow (*Dhanurasana*; see pages 55–57). The wisest course is to listen to your own body and decide for yourself whether or not you should do these postures.

## PREGNANCY

If you are pregnant, please follow the advice of your physician as to whether yoga is appropriate for you. If so, there are many excellent prenatal yoga videos and books available that show you how to modify postures for pregnancy. Prenatal yoga is designed specifically for the needs of pregnant women.

## BACK PROBLEMS AND OTHER ACHES AND PAINS

People who have suffered back injuries should exercise caution in backward bends such as The Cobra (*Bhujangasana*; see pages 49–50) and Cat-Cow (see pages 40–41). Keep in mind that the aim of backward bends is to extend the spine, not to drastically arch the back or crunch the lower spine.

In forward bends, avoid rounding your lower back, which puts pressure on your spine and can exacerbate existing back problems.

If you have any neck injuries, you should not perform Shoulder Stand (*Sarvangasana*; see pages 76–78). Instead, you may wish to do the Legs Up the Wall pose (*Viparita Karani*; see page 81).

People with high blood pressure and glaucoma should not stay in forward bends (even Standing Forward Bend; see page 44) or inversions for more than a few seconds. Again, you can replace doing a Shoulder Stand with Legs Up the Wall.

## SITTING/MEDITATIVE POSTURES
## SIMPLE SITTING POSE (*SUKHASANA*)

1. Sit cross-legged on the floor.

2. Pull the flesh of the buttocks away from the sitting bones to feel a connection to the floor.

3. Relax your legs and the backs of your knees. Feel the gentle pull of gravity on your lower body.

4. Center your pelvis. If your pelvis were a bowl of water, the water would be level.

5. Allow your spine to "grow" up to the sky.

6. Relax your shoulders back and down. Open your heart and allow your heart to lift.

7. Maintain a small arch in your lumbar (lower) spine.

8. Close your eyes and observe the inner landscape of your body and mind. Observe whatever sensations that may arise. Observe whatever thoughts that may arise.

## *Modifications*

- For weak backs, lean against the wall with a cushion on your lower back to maintain a lumbar arch.
- For uncomfortable knees, place cushions or pillows under your knees.
- If your hips feel comfortable and you're ready for a more advanced seated posture, try Diamond Pose (*Vajrasana*; page 34).

## *Benefits*

- Strengthens your lower back.
- Opens your hips.
- Allows awareness to focus inward.
- Serves as "home base."

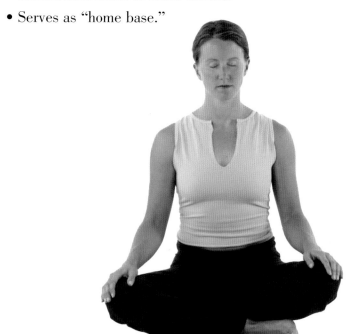

# DIAMOND POSE (VAJRASANA)

1. Kneel on the floor and sit on your heels.

2. Bring your knees together and feet together. Let your toes touch, but your heels are apart.

3. Allow your spine to lengthen up.

4. Try not to stick your ribs out or curve your lower back too much. Think about keeping the energy moving vertically through your trunk.

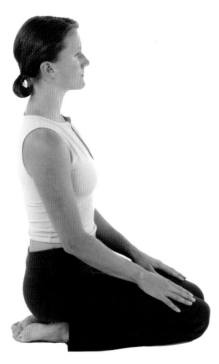

### Modifications

- If this position is mildly uncomfortable, try using a blanket under your knees and/or a rolled up blanket or pillow between your buttocks and heels.
- If this position is painful or very uncomfortable, come out of it and return to Simple Sitting Pose (*Sukhasana*; see pages 32–33).

### Benefits

- Encourages verticality in your spine and correct position of pelvis in seated postures.
- Supports the base of your spine.
- Aids digestion.
- Eases sciatica.

## WARM-UPS
### EYE MOVEMENTS/MASSAGE
### (*NETRA VYAAYAAMAM*)

1. Sit comfortably with an erect posture. Relax your shoulders and face. Have your chin parallel to the floor.

2. Keeping your head still and centered, lift your eyes up toward the ceiling (Photo A).

3. Steadily move your eyes in a straight line down toward the floor.

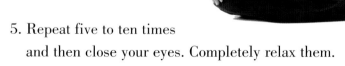

A

4. Continue this vertical eye movement, looking up and down, while keeping your breath steady. Do not focus your eyes on anything. Just feel your eye muscles stretch smoothly.

5. Repeat five to ten times and then close your eyes. Completely relax them.

6. Now open your eyes again. Keeping your head centered, make horizontal movements, back and forth from left to right, with your eyes. Move them smoothly and without focusing. Keep breathing!

7. Repeat five to seven times, then relax.

8. Open your eyes again. Look up to the ceiling and slowly move your eyes in a clockwise direction (Photo B).

9. Observe the sensations in your optic muscles. Notice where your eyes may be getting "stuck" and slow down through those spots as you breathe evenly.

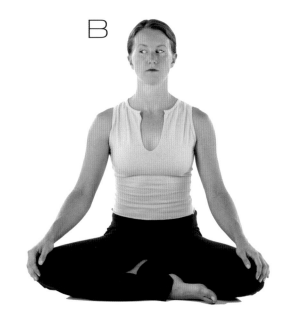

B

10. After about 15 seconds, close your eyes and relax them.

11. Open your eyes and start again in a counterclockwise direction for about 15 seconds.

12. Close your eyes and relax them. Bring your palms together in front of the heart and rub them together briskly to generate heat. (You can also blow into your palms if that helps to warm up your hands.)

13. When your palms are warm, cup them over your eyes with your fingers relaxed on your forehead. Don't apply pressure to your eyes. Allow your shoulders and face to relax. Breathe steadily, letting the warmth and darkness of your palms soothe your eyes.

14. When your palms have cooled down, allow your fingers to trickle over your closed eyes (Photo C) and then out toward your temples.

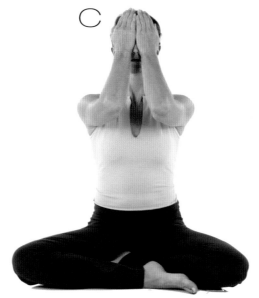

15. Massage your face, allowing your fingertips to go wherever there is tension: lightly pinch the bridge of your nose; rub your eyebrows; massage your cheeks, scalp, neck, shoulders; gently pull on your earlobes.

16. When you are finished, sit quietly with your eyes closed and observe how your eyes feel.

### *Benefits*
- Relieves fatigue and eyestrain.
- Strengthens optic nerves and muscles to prevent eye problems.
- Promotes awareness of subtle sensations, which is a good attitude to cultivate for *asana* practice.

## SHOULDER ROLLS

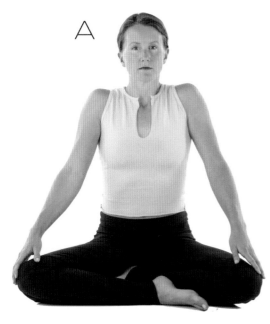

A

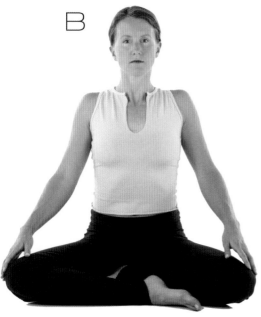

B

1. Sitting comfortably with legs crossed, inhale and bring your shoulders up to your ears (Photo A).

2. Exhale as you roll your shoulders back and down (Photo B).

3. Repeat several times.

### *Modifications*

• If your shoulders ache, or if you've had recent surgery or shoulder problems, you may want to simply shrug the shoulders up on the inhalation and let the shoulders relax down on the exhalation.

### *Benefits*

• Releases tension in the shoulders, which is where you carry the bulk of your daily stress.

• Promotes synchronization of the breath and movement, which is another thing you want to cultivate in your *asana* practice.

## THE LION (*SIMHASANA*)

1. Sit in Simple Sitting Pose (*Sukhasana*) or Diamond Pose (*Vajrasana*) with your hands on the knees (Photo A).

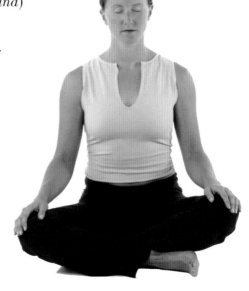

2. Inhale deeply.

3. As you exhale, lean forward, open your mouth widely, and stick your tongue all the way out down to your chin (Photo B). Roll your eyes up and let out a little "roar." (It sounds more like "ahhhh.")

4. Repeat as necessary.

### *Modifications*

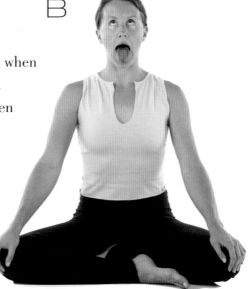

- Just the facial aspect of the Lion can be done at any point in the day when you are feeling head or eye tension. This is especially good if you've been forcing a polite smile all day.

### *Benefits*

- Relieves symptoms of TMJ (temporomandibular joint disorder) and eyestrain.
- Provides release valve for anger or frustration.

# CAT-COW

1. Come to your hands and knees. Position your hands directly under your shoulders with fingers spread out and facing forward. Align your knees directly under your hips. Gaze down at the floor.

2. Take a few breaths in this neutral position, gently lengthening your spine and neck.

3. Exhale, curl your tailbone under, round your back, and drop your head between your arms. Allow your neck to relax completely. Push your palms into the floor, keep your arms straight. This is the Cat Pose (Photo A).

4. Inhale, turn your tailbone up, arch your back gently, roll your shoulders back, and look up. This is the Cow Pose (Photo B).

5. Alternate between Cat and Cow. Allow your breath to initiate the movement.

A

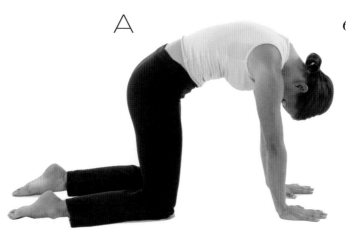

6. Breathe slowly and completely from your diaphragm up through your chest and then back. Exhale and contract your belly into your body during Cat Pose. Inhale and relax

your belly toward the floor on Cow Pose. Be careful to keep the weight on your palms, not your wrists.

7. Continue at a relaxed pace for 30–60 seconds, using the stretch as a time to investigate the sensations in your back, hips, neck, and knees. Stay with all the feelings that come up.

### *Modifications*

- If you're having back problems, be careful not to overarch your back. Think instead of lengthening your spine.
- If your wrists are sensitive, instead of placing your palms flat, make fists and bring the base of your knuckles to the floor. Face your palms in toward your body.
- If you're feeling flexible, try pointing the fingers in toward you with the heels of your hands pointing forward.

### *Benefits*

- Warms up your spine.
- Generates energy and removes energy blocks from your spine.
- Relaxes your neck and shoulders.
- Calms your nervous system.

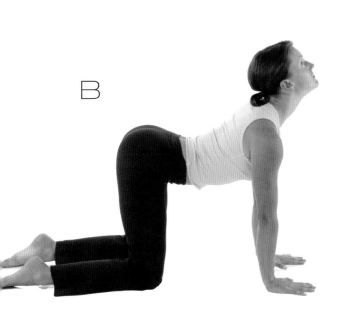

B

# SUN SALUTATION (*SURYA NAMASKAR*)

### *Position One: Mountain Pose* (Tadasana)

1. Stand with your feet together and palms together in front of your heart, thumbs resting on your sternum (Photo A).

2. Allow your shoulders to roll back and down. Lightly press your shoulder blades into the back to open your chest.

3. Feel your heart opening and lifting slightly.

4. Align your shoulders over your hips, your hips over your knees, and your knees over your ankles.

5. Feel your feet broadening and opening into the floor. Imagine that there are roots extending through your feet into the earth and revel for a moment in that connection.

6. Feel the crown of your head gracefully floating up to the sky as your whole spine is growing vertically.

7. Stay in Mountain Pose for as long as it takes to feel centered and strong. Become aware of your breath: let each inhalation "grow" you a little taller, let each exhalation relax your shoulders and face a little more. Connect with your breath and feel it enliven all the cells of your body. Become aware of your body as a whole: notice what's happening inside you, emotionally, physically, and mentally. Where are you open? Where are you closed? Tired? Awake? Numb? Enlivened? Sore? Flexible? Stiff? Comfortable? Uncomfortable? Get used to this inquiry and exploration, as it will be a part of the process of each *asana*.

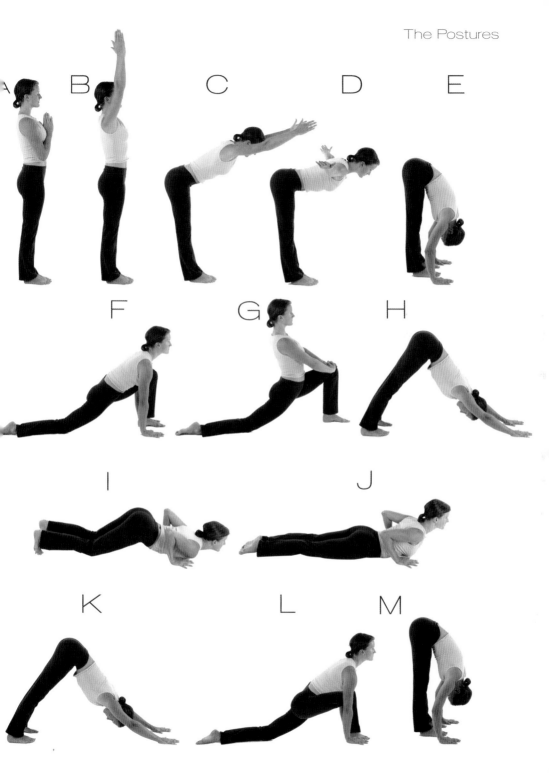

A    B    C    D    E

F    G    H

I    J

K    L    M

### *Position Two: Arms Up*

8.  On an inhalation, lift up your arms alongside your ears and bend slightly from your upper back (Photo B). To come into this position, you may reach your arms forward and up, or out to the sides and up—whichever feels more comfortable and opening to you.

### *Position Three: Forward Bend* (Uttanasana)

9.  On an exhalation, fold forward from your hips while keeping your back flat and extended. Again, you may come down with your arms extended in front of you, alongside your ears (Photo C), or with your arms out to the sides as if you're swan diving off of a diving board (Photo D). If your back needs support, try bending your knees as you fold over.

10. Once you have folded over, allow your arms to dangle (Photo E). Pretend your spine and arms are molasses, dripping slowly down. Relax your shoulders, neck, and belly. Gently shake your head "no."

11. Spread your toes and roll your weight forward slightly so that the balls of your feet are bearing most of the weight. Lift your tailbone and allow your legs to straighten, but don't lock your knees. If you're having back problems, you may choose to bend the knees slightly.

12. Breathe deeply, allowing the blood to flow to your head. Stay in your forward bend for as long as you feel comfortable. You may want to sigh loudly, flutter your lips on your exhale, or make other sounds to release your throat.

## *Position Four: Lunge*

13.  Squat down and bring your palms or fingertips to the floor outside your feet. Make sure that your fingertips and toes are lined up.

14.  Stretch your right leg as far back as it will go, and lower your right knee to the floor (Photo F). Point your right toes back with the top of your right foot on the floor. Relax your hips and pelvis and let the torso lengthen up from your hips to the crown of your head. Feel your heart lifting. (You may need to come up onto your fingertips to facilitate that lift.) Make sure that your left knee is directly over your left ankle. Don't let your knee extend past your foot. Breathe steadily and feel the way your hips are slowly opening.

14a. As you become more comfortable in the lunge, try walking your hands up to your knee and lift your torso even higher (Photo G). Then reach your arms up and lift your chest high, allowing your heart to sing and your hips to sink forward and down.

## *Position Five: Downward Facing Dog*

15.  Swing your left leg back to meet the right to make an inverted V-shape (Photo H). Your feet should be about hip distance apart. Pretend that someone is standing behind you pulling your hips back. Lift your tailbone. Press your sitting bones up and back. Bend your knees slightly, if needed. Relax your neck, broaden your shoulders away from your ears, and look back at your feet. Your heels don't have to touch the floor. Just keep pressing down with your hands, keep lifting your tailbone, and, most importantly, keep breathing steadily.

### *Position Six: Knees, Chest, Chin*

16. Keeping your hands and feet right where they are, lower your knees, chest, and chin to the floor (Photo I). Your chest and chin are between your hands and your elbows are hugging your rib cage. Lift your pelvis off the floor.

**NOTE:** If you have difficulty lowering your knees, chest, and chin down, then bring your entire body to the floor, scoot your palms to the floor underneath your shoulders, and slide your upper body back a few inches in order to lift the pelvis up.

### *Position Seven: Cobra*

17. Slide your body slightly forward (Photo J). Lower your pelvis to the floor while you lift your chest and head up *without using your hands*. Point your toes back and lengthen your upper body.

### *Position Eight: Downward Facing Dog*

18. Tuck your toes under, press your palms down, and ease your body back into Downward Facing Dog (Photo K). If this is too difficult, come onto all fours first and then lift your buttocks and hips up into Down Dog. Hold for a few seconds longer than your first Down Dog and really stretch into it. Lengthen your spine, arms, and legs. Take two or three slow, deep breaths.

### *Position Nine: Lunge*

19. Look up at your hands and swing your right foot between your hands. Bring your left knee down on the floor (Photo L). Make sure your right foot is in line with your hands. If this is too difficult, place your left knee down first and then scoop your right foot forward with your hand. Relax your hips and pelvis. Lift your heart.

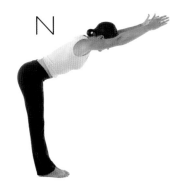

### Position Ten: Forward Bend (Uttanasana)

20. Bring your left foot forward to meet the right foot and hang in a forward bend for a breath or two to allow the spine to decompress (Photo M).

### Position Eleven: Reverse Dive

21. Reverse the movement you made coming into your forward bend in Position Three. If you had your arms by your ears (Photo N), come up the same way, or try a reverse swan dive back up. Keep your back flat during the movement. Bend your knees, if necessary. Once your arms are up alongside your ears and your body is vertical, bend back slightly from the upper back while looking up.

### Position Twelve: Mountain Pose (Tadasana)

22. Stand with your hands in prayer position in front of your heart and observe the changes in your body and mind.

23. Do three to five rounds of Sun Salutations (*Surya Namaskar*).

### Modifications

- If you are feeling sluggish and want to increase the warmth or energy in your body, do the Sun Salutation rapidly. If you are feeling anxious, perform it slowly.
- Once you are comfortable with the pattern of the Sun Salutation, try to let your breath initiate each position as follows:
  Position One: Exhale.
  Position Two: Inhale as you lift your arms.

Position Three: Exhale as you fold over.

Position Four: Inhale as you move your leg back.

Position Five: Exhale as you move into Downward Facing Dog.

Position Six: Inhale as you lower your knees, chest, and chin.

Position Seven: Hold your breath as you slide into Cobra.

Position Eight: Exhale into Downward Facing Dog and hold for three breaths.

Position Nine: Inhale into lunge.

Position Ten: Exhale into a forward bend.

Position Eleven: Inhale all the way back up.

Position Twelve: Exhale in Mountain Pose and begin the next round.

- When you've memorized the positions in the Sun Salutation, try switching the leg that goes the back in Position Four from round to round. In the first round, your right leg goes back in Position Four (and comes forward into a lunge in Position Nine). In the second round, move your left leg back. If you get confused as to which leg is supposed to come forward into the lunge in Position Nine, remember it is the same leg that you moved back in Position Four.

### *Benefits*

- Is the most complete yogic activity.
- Warms up the entire body.
- Clears energy blocks in the body.
- Soothes and focuses the mind, especially if done with great attention to the breath.

## BACKWARD BENDS

Backward bends generally stimulate your nervous system, help correct stooped posture, and help make (or keep) your spine flexible. Be sure to elongate your spine in the backbends. Think of it as one long, uninterrupted stream of energy. Do not crunch the back of your neck or lower back. To recover from one or more backbends, come into a forward bend like Child's Pose (*Balasana*; see pages 74–75).

## THE COBRA (*BHUJANGASANA*)

1. Lie down on your stomach. Relax your body completely with your face turned to the side.

2. Turn your forehead to rest on the floor. Place your palms on the floor underneath your shoulders. Line your fingertips up with your heart. Hug your elbows to your rib cage (Photo A).

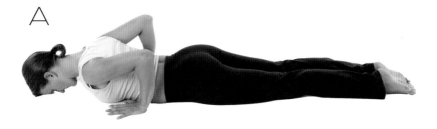

A

3. Draw your shoulder blades gently down your back toward your feet and slightly in toward each other so there's a small indentation in your upper back.

4. Bring your legs together, heels touching, and toes pointing backward.

B

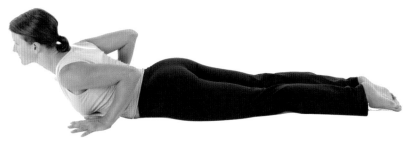

5. Inhale and slowly lift your head and shoulders, but do not press down on your hands (Photo B). Imagine that you are stretching forward and up, from your navel to the crown of your head.

6. Look up at the ceiling without crunching the back of your neck. Do not allow your neck to sink between your shoulders. Keep your legs active but not tense. Breathe naturally. Hold for 15 seconds, lower down, then repeat.

### *Modifications*
- If your back is especially stiff or inflexible, keep your forearms on the floor as you lift up comfortably.
- If your lower back hurts, separate your legs as much as you need to.
- If your back is flexible, or if your arms are particularly strong, apply a little more pressure to your palms and gradually make your arms straighter.

### *Benefits*
- Keeps your spine supple and strong.
- Strengthens your upper back.
- Tones your buttocks and lower back.
- Tones and massages your kidneys and reproductive organs.

# HALF LOCUST (ARDHA SALABHASANA)

1. Lie down on your stomach, turn your head to one side, and relax your body completely.

2. Tuck your arms underneath your body with your palms facing up against your thighs (Photo A). Keep your arms relaxed with your elbows as close together as possible.

3. Place your chin on the floor. Move your shoulders away from your ears and point your toes back.

4. Keeping all other parts of your body relaxed, draw your right foot back away from you. Inhale and lift your right leg off the floor.

5. Extend your right leg straight back behind (Photo B). Keep your foot relaxed and kneecap pointing directly down. Keep your hips square and pressing down on your arms. Try not to use the relaxed leg as leverage. Breathe steadily.

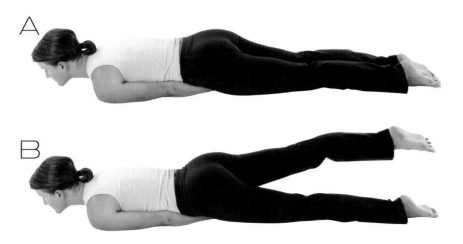

A

B

6. Hold for 10 seconds or three deep breaths. Relax your right leg down and repeat on the left side to complete one round.

7. Do another round, holding each leg for 10 seconds or three deep breaths.

### *Modifications*
- If having your arms under your body is very uncomfortable, leave your arms alongside your body with palms facing down.
- You can place a folded up blanket under your hips to avoid pressure on your hipbones.

### *Benefits*
- Strengthens your lower back, abdomen, buttocks, and legs.
- Aids digestion by putting pressure on the ascending and descending colon.
- Relieves sciatica.
- Massages your internal organs and tones your intestines, pancreas, and kidneys.

# FULL LOCUST (*SALABHASANA*)

1. Lie down on your stomach, turn your head to one side, and relax your body completely.

2. Tuck your arms underneath your body with your palms facing up against your thighs. Keep your arms relaxed with your elbows as close together as possible.

3. Place your chin on the floor. Move your shoulders away from your ears and point your toes back (Photo A).

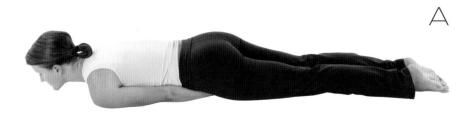

A

4. Shift your weight onto your shoulders by moving your hands closer to your knees. You can do this by tucking your toes under and pushing yourself forward. For extra leverage, you can make loose fists with your hands.

5. Extend both legs straight back. Inhale and lift them up off the ground (Photo B). Keep your legs straight and together. Keep your spine long. Don't worry about how high you are lifting your legs. The challenge is in keeping the energy moving back, not up. Breathe steadily.

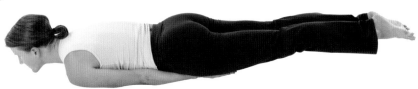

6. Hold for 10 seconds or three deep breaths.

### *Modifications*

- If having your arms underneath your body is uncomfortable, place your arms alongside your body with palms facing down. You may also want to lift your head, neck, and chest (Photo C). Keep your lower back and neck from curving back too dramatically.

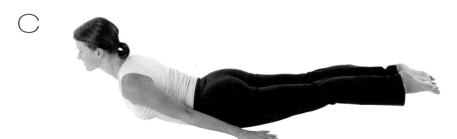

- You can place a folded blanket under your hips to ease the pressure on your hipbones.
- If keeping your legs together is a strain on your back, separate your legs or hold a folded-up towel or pillow between your legs.

### *Benefits*

- Strengthens your lower back, buttocks, and legs.
- Massages and tones your liver, intestines, pancreas, kidneys, lungs, and sympathetic nervous system.

# THE BOW (*DHANURASANA*)

1. Lie on your stomach and separate your legs so they're hip-width apart.

2. Bend your knees, bring your heels in toward your hips, and reach your hands back to grab hold of your legs wherever you can comfortably reach: the ankles, feet, toes, or pant legs (Photo A).

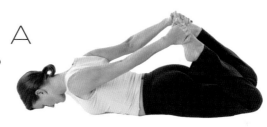

3. Rest your forehead on the floor and, for a moment, allow your entire body to relax.

4. On an inhalation, feel both halves of your body float up slowly. Lift your head, neck, chest, and knees up into the air (Photo B). Keep your arms loose and passive, like the string on a bow. Let your feet pull your shoulders back. Keep your knees and shoulders on the same level.

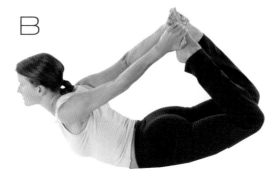

5. Look up toward the ceiling. Lift your chest, open your heart. Balance on your abdomen, not your pelvis or pubic bone.

6. Hold for about 15 seconds and float easily down. Repeat, bringing your legs a little closer together, if possible.

### *Modifications*

- If you can't reach your legs, use a strap (either a yoga strap, the belt from your bathrobe, or a rolled-up bath towel). Try not to rely on your arm strength to bring you into the pose. As the furniture movers say, "Lift with your legs."
- If lifting up off the ground is too difficult, simply remain in the preparatory pose (legs bent, hands on legs, forehead on floor) and breathe deeply, or try doing the bow on only one side of your body at a time (Photo C). (This is called Half-Bow or *Ardha Dhanurasana*.)

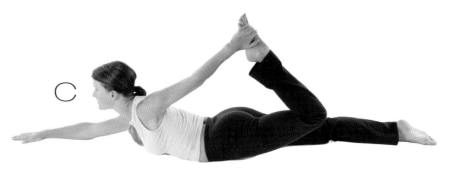

- If lifting your knees is your stumbling block, experiment with grabbing hold of different parts of your leg and see what makes lifting easier.
- If staying up is difficult, then concentrate on lifting up on the inhalation and lowering down immediately on the exhalation. Do this smoothly several times.

Yoga has amazing practical benefits when you're traveling, such as releasing tightness and stagnation from long hours of sitting. But there's also the other element of yoga: it grounds you and provides inner reflection so that you can see the constant within the diversity. It also teaches you the skill of listening to your body so that you don't push yourself to keep up your usual practice if that's not appropriate. It's best not to be overly ambitious with your practice if you're traveling. Focus on one or two things and really stay with them.

—Shiva Rea, yoga teacher, writer, workshop and retreat leader, and founder of Yogadventures

### Benefits

- Opens your chest and corrects stooping posture.
- Stretches your shoulders, hip flexors, and abdomen.
- Strengthens your legs.
- Increases flexibility of your spine.
- Relieves indigestion, gas, and constipation.
- Tones your reproductive organs.
- Stimulates your adrenal glands, energizing your body.

## THE FISH (*MATSYASANA*)

The Fish Pose (*Matsyasana*) is generally practiced as a counterpose to Shoulder Stand (*Sarvangasana*; see pages 76–78). It is held for about one-third of the time that Shoulder Stand is held.

1. Lie flat on your back. Bring your legs and feet close together. Take hold of the outsides of your thighs with your hands. Draw the elbows in close to your rib cage.

2. Rise up onto your elbows as if you were propping yourself up to look at your feet (Photo A).

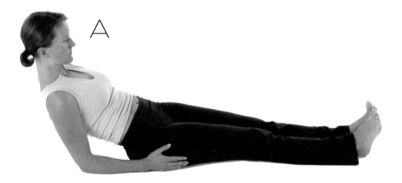

3. Move your pelvis toward your feet and lift your rib cage high up into the air. Arch your upper body. Hold on to your thighs for leverage.

4. Let your head relax back and lower the top of your head to the floor (Photo B). If the top of your head doesn't reach the floor, move your elbows closer to your feet and lift your chest a little higher. Your weight should be evenly distributed between your head, elbows, and buttocks. Your legs are energized, but not stiff.

B

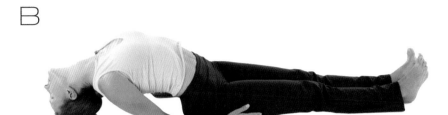

5. Close your lips. Draw the shoulders away from the ears. Relax the base of your throat and breathe deeply.

6. When you've held the pose for about a third as long as your Shoulder Stand, carefully lift your head back off the ground and roll yourself down one vertebra at a time.

7. Lie restfully on your back. Roll your head from side to side. Bend your knees and hug them into your chest. You can also interlace your fingers behind your head, cradling the back of the head as you lift your head up and stretch your neck.

### *Modifications*
- If the top of the head still cannot reach the floor, then come out of the preparatory pose. Roll up a towel or blanket and place it under your shoulder blades. Lie back over the towel and relax your head. Relax the base of your throat.
- If you are comfortable in the posture and no longer need your elbows for support, bring your hands into prayer position in front of your heart. Let your thumbs rest in your sternum and keep lifting your chest. You may then want to extend your arms away from you (Photo C).

C

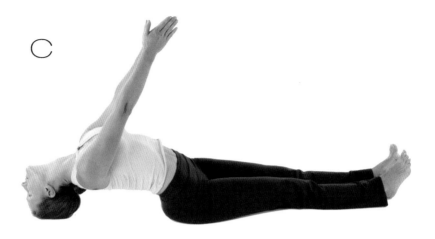

- Alternately interlace your fingers and bring the backs of your knuckles to the underside of the chin, allowing your elbows to relax out to the sides.

### Benefits
- Promotes elasticity of your lungs.
- Opens your bronchial tubes, trachea, and larynx, encouraging deep breathing and the absorption of oxygen. May relieve symptoms of asthma.
- Opens your chest, correcting bad posture habits.
- Strengthens your neck.
- Together with Shoulder Stand (*Sarvangasana*; see pages 76–78), Fish Pose tones and stimulates the thyroid and parathyroid glands in the base of your throat. Shoulder Stand stimulates the production of the hormone thyroxine and Fish Pose releases it into the blood system.
- Inverting the upper body tones your pineal and pituitary glands.

# BRIDGE POSE (*SETU BANDHASANA*)

1. Lie on your back and hug your knees into your chest.

2. Lower the soles of your feet to the floor, hip-width apart, with your heels as close to your buttocks as is comfortable (Photo A). Allow your toes, heels, and buttocks to line up. Your arms are alongside your body.

A

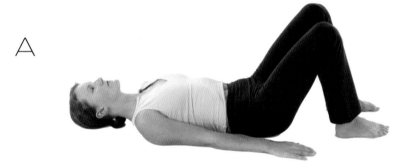

3. Exhale and press your feet and arms down. Engage your buttocks and lift your hips up toward the ceiling.

4. Bring your arms underneath your body and, if you can, interlace your fingers with your palms touching and your knuckles pointing toward your feet (Photo B).

B

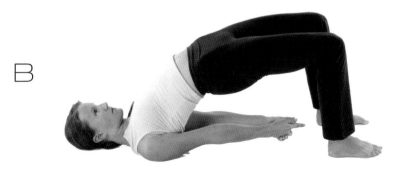

5. Keep your kneecaps pointed up toward the ceiling by actively pressing down your big toes and inner feet. Hold for 15–30 seconds, building up to 45–60 seconds.

6. Come out of the posture on an exhale, releasing your spine one vertebra at a time.

### *Modifications*

- If you can't bring your hands together underneath your body, just leave your arms parallel to the torso.
- If lifting your hips off the floor is too strenuous, try placing a large pillow, sofa cushion, or ice bucket underneath your sacrum and be passive in the posture while keeping your knees and thighs actively pressing toward each other.

### *Benefits*

- Opens your heart area and lungs.
- Tones your abdomen.
- Stimulates your thyroid.

## FORWARD BENDS

Whereas backward bends stimulate your body and mind, forward bends soothe them. The deep stretching of your spine and hamstrings releases pockets of stress in your body. The position of your head allows for blood flow to your brain, which provides a nourishing ground for the production of neuro-transmitters. The internal organs are massaged and toned, allowing for better digestion and overall functioning.

The two keys to optimal forwarding bending are: 1) to keep your spine long and not rounded and 2) to fold frontward and down from your hips, as if your hips were a hinge, rather than just plunking your upper body over your legs.

To recover from a forward bend, lie on your back with your knees hugged into your chest and breathe into your lower back.

## THE STAFF (*DANDASANA*)

The Staff is the base posture for all forward bends and spinal twists (see pages 92–97). It prepares your body for optimum forward stretching.

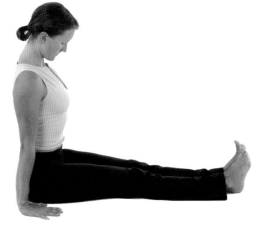

1. Sit with your legs extended in front of you, feet flexed, knees and ankles together.

2. Pull the flesh of your buttocks out from under your sitting bones so that the sitting bones are grounded.

3. Rotate your hips and pelvis forward so that your lower back is vertical and tall.

4. Place your palms on the floor next to your hips.

5. Energize the backs of your legs toward the floor.

6. Roll your shoulders back and down. Lift your sternum. Lift your rib cage and lightly engage your abdomen.

7. Tuck your chin slightly toward your chest to lengthen your cervical spine. Breathe steadily and observe your body. Continue to lengthen out through your heels and up through the crown of the head. Hold for five full and conscious breaths.

### *Modifications*

• If straightening your lower back or rotating your hips forward feels unnatural or difficult, sit on a folded blanket or pillow.
• If your hamstrings are very tight, do not completely straighten your legs. Instead, gradually work toward moving the backs of your knees toward the floor. Place a rolled-up towel under your knees for support.
• If the position is comfortable, try lifting your heels off the floor and/or lifting one leg off the floor at a time while keeping both legs strong.

### *Benefits*

• Promotes healthy posture and a nice release of tension in your hamstrings.
• Passive stretch to wrists helps relieve or prevent carpal tunnel syndrome.

# HEAD-TO-KNEE POSE (*JANUSIRSHASANA*)

1. Sit in Staff Pose (*Dandasana*): legs together and extended, feet flexed (Photo A).

2. Bend your right knee. Place the sole of your right foot on the floor and hug your right knee to your chest.

3. Open your right knee out to the side with the sole of your right foot against the inside of your left leg. If your right knee doesn't reach the floor, place a cushion beneath the knee or thigh for comfort.

4. Turn your torso to face your left leg. Your left leg is positioned directly in front of your body, not turned out to the side.

5. If your back is inflexible or the hamstrings very tight, keep your left leg bent. Otherwise, keep it straight and energized toward the floor with your left foot flexed.

6. Lift your chest, straighten your spine. Inhale, lift your arms up alongside your ears, and extend your spine forward and up.

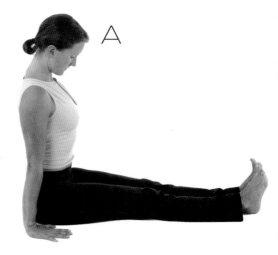

7. Exhale, fold forward from your hips, keep bringing your torso forward as if you're trying to touch your chest to your left foot. Keep your spine long and straight. Avoid rounding your back.

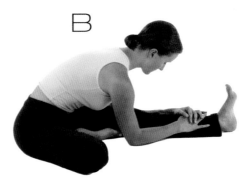

8. Take hold of your left leg with your hands at wherever your hands naturally reach. Allow your head to relax down toward your left knee (Photo B). Breathe deeply and fully while exploring the sensations in your hamstring, calf, and lower back. Aim for comfort in the pose, allowing your muscles to stretch gently.

9. Hold for 15–30 seconds. Repeat on the right side.

### *Modifications*

• If it's not possible to come all the way forward and down over your leg, or if it hurts to let your neck relax down toward your knee,

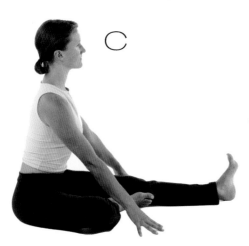

just come down and forward a few inches with a flat back and head in line with your spine (Photo C).

• Place a pillow or couch cushion on top of the leg that you will be folding over in order to rest your head.

- More-flexible people may enjoy placing the foot of the bent leg on the thigh, rather than on the inside, of the opposite leg (Photo D).

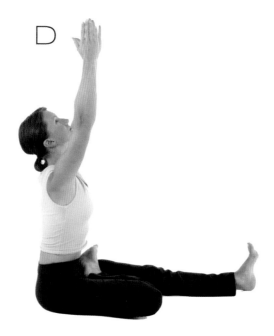

D

### *Benefits*

- Stretches your spine deeply to relieve stress in the lumbar.
- Massages internal organs.
- Opens the back of your legs and hamstrings.
- Improves flexibility.
- Relieves constipation.
- Helps control sexual energy.

# FULL FORWARD BEND
# (*PASCHIMOTANASANA*)

1. Sit in Staff Pose (*Dandasana*): legs together and extended, feet
   flexed (Photo A).

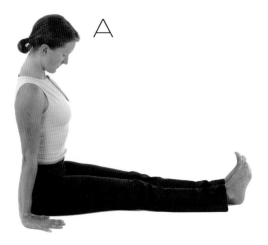

2. Inhale your arms up
   alongside your ears.
   Lifting your sternum,
   engage your abdomen.

3. Exhale, lowering your
   upper body forward
   and down over your
   legs.

4. Loosely grip whatever
   part of the leg is easily
   within reach (Photo B).
   Avoid hunching your
   shoulders or extending
   your arms farther than
   is comfortable.

5. Inhale, lifting your head
   and chest but keeping
   your hands in place.

6. Exhale and extend a little farther toward your feet. Pretend you
   are trying to touch your feet with your chest.

7. Repeat this extension as many times as you'd like to continue lengthening your spine. Eventually, allow your upper body to rest over your legs, holding the position for about 60 seconds. Completely relax your shoulders and neck. Breathe deeply and observe the sensations in your spine, hips, neck, and shoulders.

8. To release the posture, extend your arms alongside your ears and rise up with a flat back, or simply sit slowly back up while you walk your hands toward your trunk.

## *Modifications*

- If it's not possible to come all the way forward and down over your legs, or if it hurts to let your neck relax down toward your knees, just come down and forward a few inches with a flat back and your head in line with your spine.
- Place a pillow or couch cushion on top of your legs in order to rest your head once you fold over.

## *Benefits*

- Promotes healthy posture and a nice release of tension in your hamstrings.
- Stretches your spine deeply to relieve stress in the lumbar.
- Massages internal organs.
- Opens the backs of your legs and hamstrings.
- Improves flexibility.
- Relieves constipation.
- Helps control sexual energy.

## COW FACE POSE (*GOMUKHASANA*)

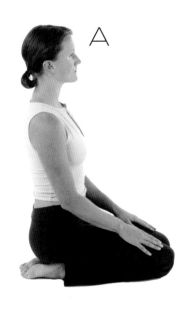

1. Begin in Diamond Pose: Kneel on the floor and sit on your heels (Photo A).

2. Shift your hips over to the right side. Keeping your legs bent, cross your left leg over your right. Ground your sitting bones and lengthen your spine.

3. As you inhale, raise up your right arm alongside your ear. Bend your arm at the elbow and reach your fingers down towards your shoulder blade (Photo B). Reach behind the back with your left arm and take hold of the fingers of the right hand (Photo C). (If your hands do not meet, see Modifications.)

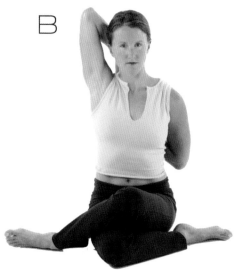

4. Inhale as you draw your shoulder blades toward each other, opening your heart. On the next inhalation, draw your shoulders down away from your ears. Hold for three to five deep breaths.

5. On an exhale, release your arms. Reverse your legs, reverse your arms, and repeat on the opposite side.

### *Modifications*

- If your hands don't meet behind your back, use a towel or strap, or simply grab hold of your shirt with each hand (Photo D).
- If your hips are tight, or it's very uncomfortable to sit with your legs bent, try remaining in Diamond Pose and just perform the arm positions.

### *Benefits*

- Loosens your shoulders.
- Opens your hips.
- Relieves tension in upper body and neck.

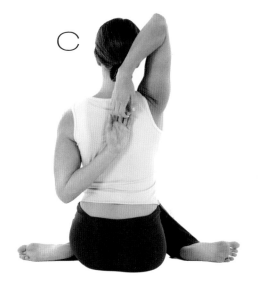

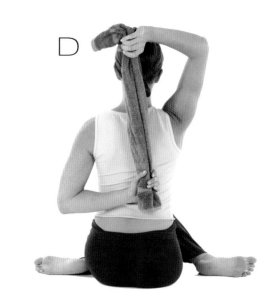

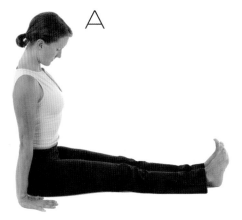

A

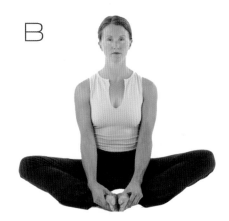

B

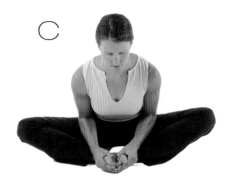

C

# BOUND ANGLE
## (*BADDHA KONASANA*)

1. Sit in Staff Pose (*Dandasana*): legs together and extended, feet flexed (Photo A).

2. Bring the soles of your feet together and draw your heels in toward you. How close your heels come in depends on your comfort level.

3. Loosely hold your toes, ankles, or shins (Photo B). Relax your knees out to the sides.

4. Continue to lengthen your spine up toward the ceiling while moving your shoulder blades down your back. Relax your hips and allow your pelvis to rotate forward.

5. If you are comfortable in this position, slowly lower your upper body forward and down with a straight back (Photo C). If you can't move your upper body forward and down without

rounding your back, then just keep your spine vertical and concentrate on letting your spine grow upward.

6. Explore the sensations in your hips and inner thighs. Allow each exhalation to relax your hips and legs even more. Hold for about 30 seconds.

## *Modifications*
- If straightening your lower back or rotating your pelvis forward feels unnatural or difficult, sit on a folded blanket or pillow.
- If sitting up tall is a problem, try coming into this posture with your back flat against the wall.
- If your knees don't reach the floor, place pillows, rolled-up towels, or blankets underneath them for support.

## *Benefits*
- Stretches your spine deeply to relieve stress in the lumbar.
- Opens your hips from their usually tight sitting position.
- Stretches your inner thighs.
- Creates space in your pelvis.
- Good for menstrual difficulties and indigestion.

# CHILD'S POSE (*BALASANA*)

1. Come to your hands and knees. Lengthen your spine. Reach your sitting bones slightly up.

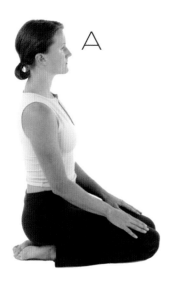

2. Sit back on your heels in Diamond Pose (*Vajrasana*; Photo A). Consciously lengthen your spine and arms.

3. Lower your forehead to the floor (Photo B). Release your neck, shoulders, upper back, middle back, and lower back. Allow your shoulders to broaden. Breathe deeply from your lower abdomen. Surrender your worries to the floor and allow your mind to stay focused on your breath.

4. For the full experience of surrendering, place your hands back by your feet with your palms facing up.

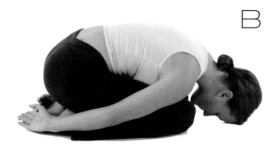

### *Modifications*
- If your buttocks don't reach your heels, try elevating your forehead with a pillow, cushion, or your hands.

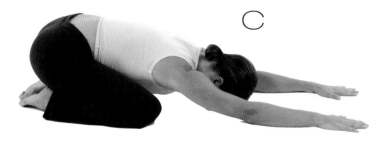

- If your back aches, sit with your knees wider apart.
- Experiment with reaching your arms out in front of you in Extended Child's Pose (Photo C).

**Benefits**
- Opens tight hips and shoulders.
- Calms your mind.
- Encourages a sense of surrender.
- Relaxes your back.
- Provides a counterpose for backward bending postures.

## INVERSIONS

An inversion is any posture where your head is lower than your hips, such as Standing Forward Bend (*Uttanasana*) and Downward Facing Dog in Sun Salutation (*Surya Namaskar*). Inversions momentarily reverse the effects of gravity on your vital organs (heart, lungs, liver, kidney, spleen, intestines, gall bladder, bladder, and stomach). They stimulate and tone them, and encourage their proper placement. In addition, inversions stimulate blood and lymph circulation, and bring fresh supplies of blood to your brain. Each separate inversion has its own unique benefits as well.

# SHOULDER STAND (*SARVANGASANA*)

Shoulder Stand puts pressure on your neck. If you have a sore neck, or very tight shoulders, you may want to opt for the Legs Up the Wall posture (*Viparita Karani*; see page 81).

You may also want to consider this alternate posture if you have high blood pressure, glaucoma, or a headache. Women who are menstruating may also opt for Legs Up the Wall instead.

Before coming into Shoulder Stand, you may want to cough or clear your throat so you won't need to while you're in the posture.

1. Lie on your back with your shoulder blades flat on the floor. Have your arms alongside your body with palms facing down. Make sure you have room behind your head for your legs.

2. Inch your shoulder blades in toward each other. Then inch your elbows in toward each other.

3. Press on your palms and lift your legs up to 90°. Then shoot your legs overhead so that they are as close to parallel to the floor as is comfortable for you (Photo A).

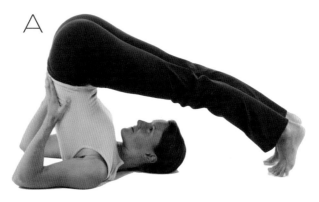

A

4. Bring your hands to your back for support.

5. Inch your shoulder blades a little closer together. Do the same for your elbows.

6. Lift your legs up toward the ceiling.

7. Once you feel settled, make your body more vertical by walking your hands closer to your shoulders and moving your pelvis closer to your face (Photo B). Relax your feet.

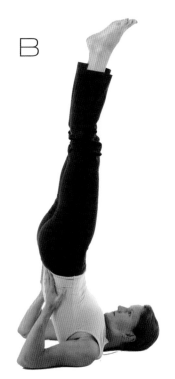

See how much you can relax without losing the posture: allow energy to circulate through your whole body.

8. Bring your chest toward your chin and feel your chin massaging the base of your throat. Hold the posture for 1–5 minutes. Remain as quiet and still as you can to benefit from the restfulness of the pose. If you need to adjust your body at all, do so mindfully, gently, and without making sudden or jarring movements.

9. To release the posture, bring the legs down so they're parallel to the floor again. Release your palms to the floor and roll down one vertebra at a time.

10. Follow this posture with its counterpose, The Fish (*Matsyasana*; see pages 58–60).

## *Modifications*

- If your neck feels uncomfortable, fold up a blanket until it is 1 to 2 inches (2.5 to 5 cm) thick. Place the blanket under your shoulders. Your head and neck should be completely off the blanket.
- If you are feeling tired or overwhelmed, or you can't easily get your legs back over your head, then try doing your Shoulder Stand against the wall (see pages 79–80).

## *Benefits*

- Releases tension in your cervical spine.
- Releases the hormone thyroxine into the blood stream, which helps to regulate all the systems of your body.
- Rests the heart (which temporarily doesn't need to work against gravity) and legs.
- Nourishes the nerves in your spine.
- Tones the abdomen when you come into and out of the pose.

# SHOULDER STAND AGAINST THE WALL

1. Sit in a comfortable Staff Pose (*Dandasana*)—legs together and extended, feet flexed—with one hip against the wall.

2. Swing your legs up along the wall and bring your back onto the floor, resting in an L shape (Photo A). Bring your buttocks as close to the wall as possible.

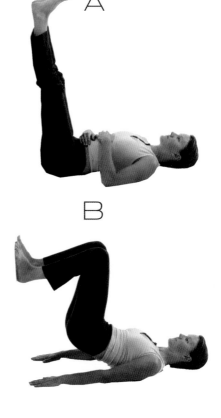

3. Bend your knees and place the soles of your feet on the wall.

4. Pressing the wall with your feet, lift your hips and pelvis up (Photo B). Keep lifting until your torso is parallel with the wall.

5. Bend your elbows and place your hands on your back for support. Little by little, bring your shoulder blades toward each other and move your shoulders away from your ears.

6. Keep your legs bent until you are ready to make your legs vertical. Straighten one leg and then the other (Photo C). Hold the pose for 1–5 minutes.

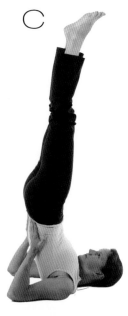

7. Release the pose by bringing your feet to the wall and then releasing your buttocks back down to the floor. Rest for a moment with your legs on the wall. Then softly roll out of the posture.

### *Modifications*

- If your neck feels uncomfortable, fold up a blanket until it is 1 to 2 inches (2.5 to 5 cm) thick. Place the blanket about a foot (30 cm) away from the wall so that it will be flush with the tops of your shoulders when you release your upper body down.

### *Benefits*

- Releases tension in your cervical spine.
- Releases the hormone thyroxine into the blood stream, which helps to regulate all the systems of your body.
- Rests the heart (which temporarily doesn't need to work against gravity) and legs.
- Nourishes the nerves in your spine.
- Tones the abdomen when you come into and out of the pose.

# LEGS UP THE WALL (*VIPARITA KARANI*)

This is a good alternate posture to Shoulder Stand if you have a sore neck, tight shoulders, high blood pressure, glaucoma, or a headache. Women who are menstruating may also want to do this posture instead.

1. Sit in a comfortable Staff Pose (*Dandasana*)—legs together and extended, feet flexed—with one hip against the wall.

2. Swing your legs up along the wall and bring your back onto the floor, resting in an L shape (Photo A). Bring your buttocks as close to the wall as possible.

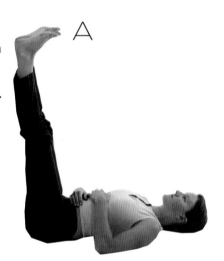

3. Stay connected to the moment by keeping your awareness on your breath. Breathe from your diaphragm up through your chest and then down.

### *Modifications*
- If you'd like more support, start the posture with a folded-up blanket under your buttocks so that when your legs are up the wall, the blanket will be positioned under your lower back.
- To release your hips, spend half of the time in the posture with the soles of the feet together (Bound Angle Pose against the wall).

### *Benefits*
- Soothes tired or aching feet and legs.
- Quiets the mind.

## STANDING POSTURES

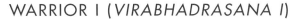

Standing postures build physical endurance and strong mental focus. By establishing a well-aligned and mindful Mountain Pose (*Tadasana*; see page 42), you can move your limbs easily into the following postures.

### WARRIOR I (*VIRABHADRASANA I*)

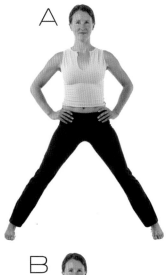

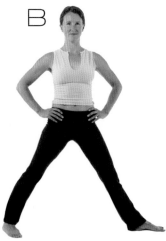

1. Stand in Mountain Pose (*Tadasana*): feet together and palms together in front of your heart. Allow your feet to broaden and open into the floor.

2. Widen your legs as securely as you can stand into a straddle position (Photo A).

3. Turn your left foot out 90° and your right foot in about 30° (Photo B). Try to line up your heels. Reconnect your feet to the floor and duplicate their openness in Mountain Pose.

4. Bend your left knee as much as you can, but don't let it go past your foot. It should be in line with your ankle.

5. Look down at your left foot. If you can't see your big and second toes, open your knee out to the left until you can.

6. Turn your hips and upper body to the left (Photo C). Do your best to square your hips and shoulders toward your left knee.

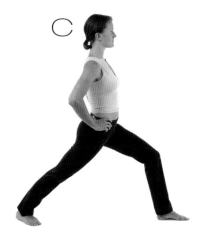

7. Press your outer right foot into the floor and keep your right leg (the back leg) strong and straight. Resist the common tendency to put all the weight on your front (bent) leg. Keep your weight evenly distributed between both feet.

8. Raise your arms up alongside your ears (Photo D). Relax your shoulders down. You may keep your arms parallel to each other or bring your palms together for an extra challenge. If your palms are together, direct your gaze at your thumbs. Otherwise, keep the gaze forward.

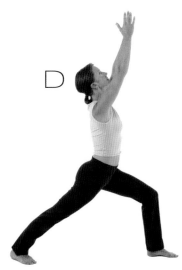

9. As you inhale, feel the lift in your heart and the elongation of your torso. As you exhale, feel your lower body pulling down toward the floor. Start by holding for 15–30 seconds and build up to holding for 45–60 seconds. Repeat on the right side.

## Modifications

• If the posture is difficult to hold, press your back heel against the wall.

- If you have high blood pressure and would rather not raise your arms higher than your heart, just bring your hands to your hips. Let your hands suggest to your hips that they want to stay squared and facing your bent knee.

### Benefits
- Strengthens your thighs, buttocks, calves, and arms.
- Opens your chest.
- Inspires a feeling of bravery and self-sufficiency.

## WARRIOR II (*VIRABHADRASANA II*)

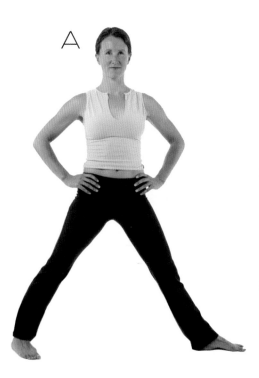

A

1. Stand in Mountain Pose (*Tadasana*): feet together and palms together in front of your heart. Be aware of the alignment of your body. Have your shoulders over your hips over your knees over your ankles. Tuck your tailbone slightly under.

2. Widen your stance and turn your feet as in Warrior I: turn your left foot out 90° and your right foot in about 30° (Photo A).

3. Bend your left knee over your left middle toes. Keep both feet strongly pressed into the floor, weight evenly distributed.

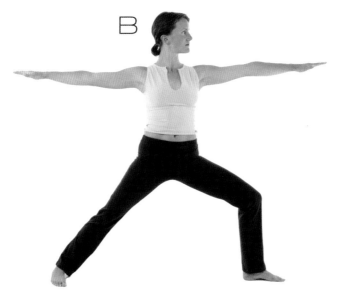

4. Instead of rotating your body toward your bent knee, as in Warrior I, keep your hips and chest open. Extend your arms out to the sides, parallel to the floor, with palms facing down (Photo B). Keep your shoulders relaxed.

5. Turn to gaze over your left fingertips. As you inhale, feel your rib cage growing vertically. As you exhale, move your hands in opposition to each other, opening your heart. Hold for 15–30 seconds, working up to 45 seconds. Repeat on the right side.

### *Modifications*
• If your legs are not developed, experiment with the span of your legs. Try narrowing the space between your feet and see if that is easier to hold until you build up your legs to a wider stance.

### *Benefits*
• Strengthens your thighs, buttocks, calves, and arms.
• Opens your shoulders, chest, and hips.
• Inspires a feeling of bravery and self-sufficiency.

# TRIANGLE (*TRIKONASANA*)

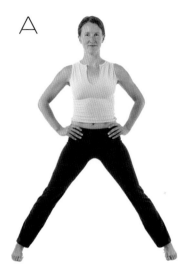

A

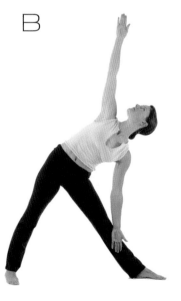

B

1. Stand in Mountain Pose (*Tadasana*): feet together and palms together in front of your heart. Relax your feet and hips.

2. Widen your legs as much as in the other Warrior postures (Photo A): 3–4 feet (91–122 cm).

3. Turn your left toes out 90°, right toes in 30°. Align your left heel with your right instep.

4. Extend your arms out to the sides, parallel to the floor, with palms facing down.

5. Look over your left fingertips and glide over to the left, shifting your hips to the left.

6. Keeping your arms straight, tilt your upper body down to the left. Lower your left hand down toward your left leg. Raise your right arm up toward the ceiling (Photo B). Rest your left hand on your left leg. Try not to bend at the waist or lock your knees. Keep your body in one plane, as if you were practicing between two screens set only a foot apart.

7. Inhale and lengthen your spine. Exhale and turn to look up at your right hand.

8. Inhale and rotate your right hip back and open. Exhale and move your hands away from each other, opening your heart.

9. Hold for 15–30 seconds. Repeat on the right side.

## *Modifications*

- If you feel unstable, experiment with the rotation of your back foot and with the distance between your legs. You may also want to practice Triangle Pose against a wall. This will also encourage keeping the body in one plane.
- If your knees are sensitive or weak, try keeping your front leg bent slightly.
- Experiment with the placement of your lower hand. Start by resting your hand on your thigh, then your shin, your ankle, and finally the floor. See how low you can place your hand without sacrificing the straightness and length of your torso.

## *Benefits*

- Opens your hips, chest, and rib cage.
- Soothes your lower back.
- Strengthens your legs and arms.
- Promotes overall balance and relaxation in your hips.

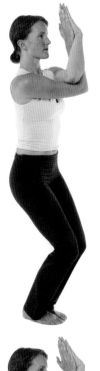

A

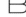

B

# EAGLE POSTURE (*GARUDASANA*)

1. Stand in Mountain Pose (*Tadasana*): feet together and palms together in front of your heart.

2. Raise your arms above your head. As you lower them, swing your right arm underneath your left arm.

3. Intertwine your forearms and bring your palms together with thumbs toward your face (Photo A).

4. Lift your elbows up to shoulder height. Move your elbows forward and feel your shoulders widening.

5. Bend your knees deeply as if you were sitting on a chair. Hoist your right leg over your left (Photo B). Relax your left foot. If you can, wrap your right foot back around your left calf.

6. As you inhale, feel your torso lengthening. Keep your chest and elbows lifted, chin parallel to the floor.

7. Try to line up your elbows over your knees, over your ankles. Find something stationary

One of the things that distinguishes yoga from other forms of physical exercise is that it is so portable. You don't need equipment like a bicycle or weights. You even barely need clothes! And it doesn't take up much space. That's why it is such a good travel companion.

—Julie Rusk, M.Ed., LPC, author of *Desktop Yoga* (Perigee), stress management expert, president of Wholesome Resources

in front of you at eye level and become one with the stillness of that object. Hold for 15 seconds. Repeat on the other side: left arm under right, left leg over right.

### Modifications
- If it's hard to line up your palms, try interlacing your fingers to bring your palms closer together.
- If you feel wobbly, focus on squeezing your legs and arms together and bending your knees a little deeper.
- If you have bad knees, you may want to focus only on the upper-body part of your posture.

### Benefits
- Improves flexibility of your hips, knees, and ankles.
- Brings fresh blood to the kidneys and reproductive organs.
- Improves focus.

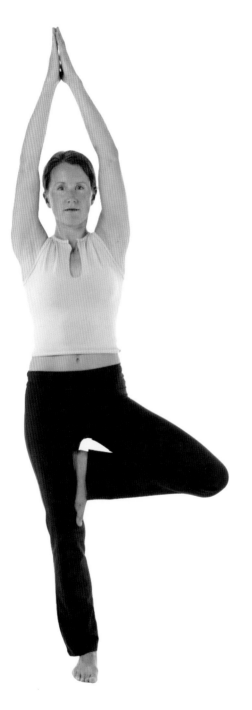

# TREE (*VRKSASANA*)

1. Stand in Mountain Pose (*Tadasana*): feet together and palms together in front of your heart.

2. Shift the weight of your body over to your right foot. Allow that foot to open to the floor with your weight distributed evenly from back to front.

3. Mindfully lift your left foot off the floor and place the sole of your left foot comfortably anywhere on the inside of the right leg: your ankle, your calf, or your inner thigh.

4. Breathe as you gradually open your left knee out to the left, opening your hips.

5. Slowly bring your hands into prayer position in front of your heart. If you are feeling stable, try raising your arms above your head either with prayer hands or separated.

6. Find a stationary object at which to gaze and mentally meld with. Pretend you are still in Mountain Pose (*Tadasana*): keep your hips level and your tailbone slightly tucked under. Allow your inhalations to lengthen your torso without sticking your ribs out. Allow your exhalations to relax your shoulders back and down. Hold for 20 seconds, building up to 45 seconds.

7. Very slowly and watchfully, release your left leg down and relax your arms. Gently shake out your arms and legs. Repeat on your right side.

### *Modifications*
- Balancing postures teach patience and self-acceptance. If you fall out of the Tree, bless yourself and get right back up. Don't be embarrassed to use a wall for support and simply focus on relaxing your hips and keeping your posture erect.

### *Benefits*
- Opens your hips, chest, and shoulders.
- Increases concentration, poise, and body awareness.
- Strengthens your legs.

## SPINAL TWISTS

Spinal twists literally squeeze your internal organs, cleansing them and filling them, on release, with a fresh supply of blood. They increase the flexibility of your spine and relieve tension in your shoulders, neck, and hips. They are invigorating. The key to a cleansing, rejuvenating twist is to lengthen your spine first and then turn.

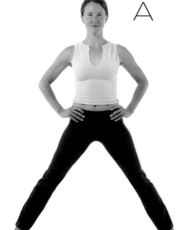

A

### STANDING SPINAL TWIST

1. Stand in Mountain Pose (*Tadasana*): feet together and palms together in front of your heart.

2. Widen your legs about 3–4 feet (91–122 cm). Keep your feet parallel and allow the soles of your feet to open to the floor (Photo A).

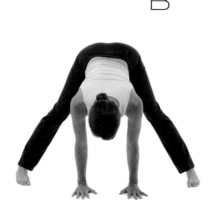

B

3. With your hands on your hips, and keeping a flat back, fold forward from your hips. Relax your torso down toward the floor.

4. Reach your hands to the floor positioned underneath your shoulders (Photo B). Flatten your palms if you can. If you can't, see "Modifications."

5. Keeping your palms on the floor, inhale as you lengthen up your torso.

6. Center your left palm. On the next inhalation, raise your right arm up toward the ceiling (Photo C). Look up at your right hand, breathing into the spinal twist. Inhale, lengthen your spine, exhale, and twist a little more.

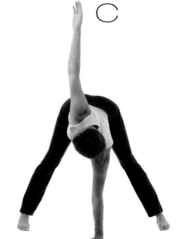

7. Release down and reverse your twist. Repeat twice more on each side, holding for a few breaths each time.

8. To release out of the pose, bring your hands back to your hips and come up with a flat back. Hop or step your feet together.

### *Modifications*
- If your hands don't reach the floor, rest your left hand on the outside of your right leg, or wherever you can comfortably reach, and reverse accordingly.
- If your hamstrings are flexible, try the posture with your legs together.

### *Benefits*
- Combines the benefits of an inversion and a spinal twist.
- Keeps your spine flexible.
- Relieves fatigue.

# SUPINE SPINAL TWIST (*JATHARA PARIVARTANASANA*)

A

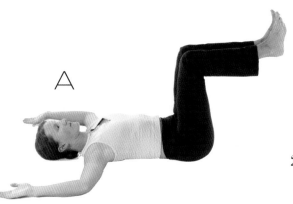

B

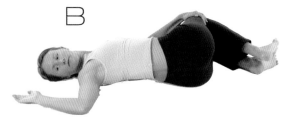

1. Lie on your back and extend your arms out to the sides at shoulder height with palms facing up. Relax your shoulders on the floor with the shoulder blades flat. Bring your knees up (Photo A).

2. Tuck your knees toward your chest and then lower them to the left. Look over your right shoulder (Photo B). Relax your body completely. Try to keep both shoulders on the floor even if it means your knees rise up a little. Hold passively for 20–30 seconds.

3. On an inhalation, lift your knees back to center and center your head. Exhale and reverse the twist.

### *Modifications*

- If rotating your head to the side is painful, keep your head centered and focus on the twist in your lower body.
- If you'd like to intensify this twist, cross one leg over the other and lower your knees in the direction of your lower leg (Photo C).

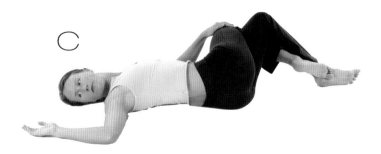

### *Benefits*

- Keeps your spine flexible.
- Relaxes your lower back.
- Relieves any backaches from sitting.
- Quiets the mind.

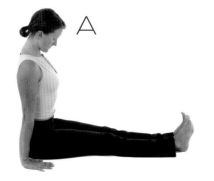

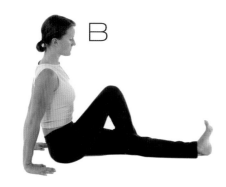

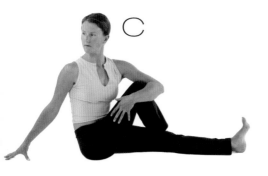

## HALF SPINAL TWIST
## (*ARDHA MATSYENDRASANA*)

1. Sit in Staff Pose (*Dandasana*):
   legs together and extended, feet
   flexed (Photo A). Bring a special
   awareness to the elongation of
   your spine.

2. Bend your right knee. Cross your
   right foot over your left leg
   (Photo B). Plant your right foot
   down with your right kneecap
   facing upward. Keep your left
   foot flexed.

3. Hug your right knee with your
   left arm (Photo C). Bring your
   right arm back behind you with
   your palm on the floor near the
   base of your spine.

4. Slowly twist to the right from
   your lower spine to your middle
   spine to your shoulders. Twist
   your neck to the right and look
   over your right shoulder. Imagine
   a line from the crown of the
   head to the tailbone and twist on
   that axis.

5. Inhale as you make yourself taller. Exhale as you twist some more. Keep your belly relaxed and allow the twist to squeeze your digestive organs. Keep your chest open; if you start to cave in, ease up on the twist and sit up straighter. Try not to lean back on the hand that's behind your back. Think of it as a second spine.

6. Hold for 20–30 seconds and release slowly. Release your legs and come back into Staff Pose (*Dandasana*) to rebuild the twist from the left.

## *Modifications*

• Establish the twist with the arm hugging the opposite knee. If it feels like you could intensify the twist without sacrificing comfort or the openness of your chest, then bring your hugging elbow to the outside of the knee. Use the elbow as a lever (Photo D).

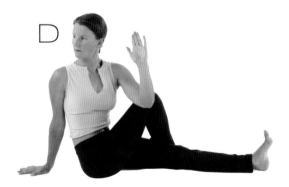

## *Benefits*

• Tones and cleanses all your vital organs.
• Keeps your spine flexible, supple, and young.
• Stimulates your adrenal glands, energizing your body.

## DEEP RELAXATION

Even with the most "inward" intentions, *asana* still focuses on the physical aspect of your life. In addition to your *asana* practice, you need time to unwind and go deeply within, to contact your more subtle self, and let go of the outside world. When you travel, it's especially important to keep in contact with that part of you that is not affected by the constantly changing surroundings. That's what nourishes you for your travels.

Corpse Pose (*Savasana*) is the basic posture of release for your body. It is an essential *asana* because it teaches you how to let go and focus on the inner experience of your body. Try to come into Corpse Pose for a few breaths between postures as well as at the end of your session.

Yogic Sleep (*Yoga Nidra*) is a deeply restful experience which takes you through the various layers of your being, from the physical to mental to spiritual. You don't have to believe in a higher self in order for the benefits of Yogic Sleep to shine through you. For the best results, try making a tape of yourself (or someone with a melodious voice) reading the instructions for Yogic Sleep.

## CORPSE POSE (*SAVASANA*)

1. Lie down on your back. Gently roll your head from side to side a few times and then center it. Tuck your chin slightly toward your chest to lengthen your neck.

2. Turn your palms faceup. Allow your legs to relax about hip-width apart or more. Flatten your shoulder blades on the floor.

3. Close your eyes and observe your breath. Scan your body and notice all its sensations. Observe the areas of tension and either

release them or accept them. Check in on how you're feeling. Allow your mind to stay alert and focused on this moment.

### *Modifications*

- For aching backs, place a rolled-up blanket or cushion under your knees, or bend your legs with the soles of your feet on the floor and knees relaxing in toward each other.
- For menstrual discomfort, have the soles of your feet touching, your knees relaxed out away from each other, and your legs in a diamond shape on the floor.
- Try to come into Relaxation Pose (*Savasana*) for a few breaths between other postures.
- Place an eye pillow or folded washcloth over your eyes to relieve eyestrain.

### *Benefits*

- Provides relaxation for your body and mind.
- Allows your awareness to center on more subtle feelings.
- Provides rest between postures and at the end of a session.

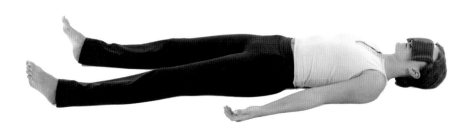

## YOGIC SLEEP (YOGA NIDRA)

Yogic Sleep takes the mind to a receptive state, so it is a good time to work on any affirmations or resolutions. Before you start the process of relaxation, think of one affirmation and resolve to plant it in your mind later. Some examples are "I am a patient and relaxed traveler" or "I am at home wherever I am."

1. Lie down on your back. It is better to lie on the floor than on a bed to prevent dozing off. You may want to have a blanket over you, or put on a sweater and socks, as your body temperature usually goes down during deep relaxation.

2. Center your head. Allow your legs to relax about hip-width apart or more. Flatten your shoulder blades.

3. Make fists with your hands. Squeeze your arms, feet, legs, buttocks, and face. Then lift everything up off the floor. Hold for a few seconds and then let everything drop.

4. Bring your awareness to your legs. Loosen them up by rolling them from side to side. Rotate your ankles a few times and then let your legs be very still.

5. Shake out your fingers and loosen up your arms. Then let them lie still on the floor.

6. Shrug your shoulders up toward your ears and then let them go. Move your shoulders down toward your feet and then let go. Move your shoulder blades together behind your back and then let go. Move your shoulders toward each other in front of your

chest and then let go. Turn your palms faceup and relax your arms.

7.  Without lifting your head, tuck your chin slightly toward your chest to lengthen your neck. Roll your head slowly from side to side and then let it settle.

8.  Move your jaw up and down, side to side, in circles, and then let it go. Press your lips together and puff out your cheeks. Pretend you've got mouthwash, swish it around, and then let it go. Suck your cheeks in and then let go.

9.  Move all your facial muscles toward your nose. Hold and release. Open your eyes widely, open your mouth widely, and stick your tongue out. Roar like a lion. Then relax your face and close your eyes.

10. Feel your body melting into the floor. Inhale into your belly and puff it out, taking in more and more breath. Hold your breath, then open your mouth and let the air gush out.

11. Inhale into your chest, letting the chest expand bigger and bigger until it cannot expand any more. Hold your breath. Let it gush out through your mouth.

12. Make whatever adjustments you need with your clothing or body, and then lie completely still. Allow your awareness to encompass your whole body and be open to its sensations, rhythms, and feelings. Allow your awareness to light on any part of the body that needs your attention.

13. Draw your awareness down to your toes. Observe the sensations there and let your toes relax.

14. Draw your awareness down to the soles of your feet. Observe the sensations there and let them relax completely.

15. Observe your ankles; relax them. Observe your calves and shins; relax them. Observe the backs of your knees; let them soften. Observe your kneecaps; relax them. Observe your thighs; relax your hamstrings, inner thighs, and quadriceps. Observe your buttocks; let them relax.

16. Observe your hips. Allow them to sink into the floor. Relax your pelvis and abdomen. Observe the sensations in your hips, pelvis, and abdomen.

17. Feel your tailbone sinking into the floor. Release your lower back; observe the sensations there. Relax your middle back; observe the sensations there. Relax your upper back and shoulder blades; observe the sensations there.

18. Feel the back of your neck releasing. Observe its sensations. Feel your upper shoulders releasing. Feel your upper arms relaxing. . .feel the crooks of your elbows softening. . .feel your forearms and wrists relax. . .feel your thumbs and fingers relax. . . feel your palms and the backs of your hands relax; observe your arms on the floor and all the sensations there.

19. Notice your solar plexus. Feel your rib cage relax. Observe your lungs. Relax your chest, feel your heart softening; observe the sensations in your chest.

20. Feel the base of your throat relax. Feel your entire throat soft-ening. Feel the roof of your mouth relax. Release the base of your tongue. Relax your jaw completely. Observe the sensations in your throat and mouth.

21. Relax your scalp and the crown of your head. Relax your fore-head, temples, and eyebrows. Relax the bridge of your nose... your nose...your cheeks...your upper lip...your lower lip... your chin; observe the sensations in your head and face. Relax your ears.

22. Scan your body and notice any areas that feel like they are still "holding on." Know that it's OK to let go completely.

23. Focus your awareness on your breath. Witness it coming and going out of your body—how your chest rises and falls and how your lungs fill. Notice how effortless it is. Witness all this for about a minute.

24. With the same attitude of witnessing, bring your awareness to the thoughts in your mind. Listen and watch your thoughts come and go like passing clouds. Observe your thoughts without becoming involved with them for about a minute.

25. Remember the affirmation or resolve that you chose before you began your Yogic Sleep and silently repeat it a few times. Don't worry if your mind conjures up resistance to the affirmation. Just let those thoughts go.

26. Observe the stillness inside you. Become aware of the gaps between your thoughts. Keep your awareness open and diffuse.

Allow your mind to be awake even as your body sleeps. Rest in this stillness for about 5 minutes.

27. Bring your awareness back to your breath. Gradually and without strain, deepen your breath. Breathe through your lower abdomen up to your chest.

28. Gently move your fingers and toes, ankles and wrists. Stretch your body. Bend your knees into your chest and roll over to your right side, resting in a fetal position for a few breaths.

29. Slowly come back to a seated position, bringing the head up last. Whenever you can, follow Yogic Sleep with breathing exercises (see below) and meditation (see Chapter Five).

## BREATHING EXERCISES (PRANAYAMA)

Your breath, mind, and body are delicately interwoven so that by changing one, you influence the others. *Pranayama* (a Sanskrit word that can be translated as "expanding the life force") is the science of breathing consciously in order to slow down, calm, and refine your mind. The three breathing exercises below can be used at any point in your day, but they work especially well when done in sequence before meditation.

### DEEP THREE-PART BREATH
### (*DIRGA SWASAM PRANAYAMA*)

1. Sit cross-legged on the floor with buttocks flesh pulled away from your sitting bones. Allow your spine to "grow" up to the sky.

2. Close your lips and begin breathing only through your nose. Allow the inhalation to expand your lower abdomen, then your rib cage, then your upper chest. Imagine that you are filling a glass with water: the bottom gets filled first, then the middle, then the top.

3. On the exhalation, relax your chest, relax your rib cage, and gently contract your abdomen in toward your spine.

4. Continue at a pace that feels comfortable for you, inhaling deeply from bottom to middle to top, exhaling slowly and completely from top to middle to bottom.

### *Modifications*
- If you are heavily congested, do your best but don't strain.

### *Benefits*
- Allows your lungs to expand to their full capacity, increasing elasticity.
- Brings up to seven times more oxygen into your bloodstream, nourishing the cells of your body.
- Allows toxins to be released on the exhalation.
- Helps to normalize blood pressure.
- Triggers relaxation response in your body.
- Allows buried emotions to surface for healing.

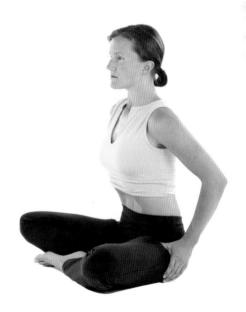

# RAPID DIAPHRAGMATIC BREATHING (*KAPALABHATI*)

1. Exhale energetically through your nose as if you are blowing out a candle with your nostrils. At the same time, lift your diaphragm and abdomen up into your rib cage.

2. Relax your diaphragm and allow the inhalation to happen passively. Repeat these two steps at a pace that feels comfortable to you.

3. After 30–60 seconds, exhale all the breath from your lungs, then take a Deep Three-Part inhalation, then exhale again, allowing your breath to return to normal. A typical pace would be one exhalation per second. Do three rounds of Rapid Diaphragmatic Breathing (*Kapalabhati*) for 30–60 seconds per round.

### *Modifications*
• If you are congested, or if you feel dizzy, simply stop and go back to doing Deep Three-Part Breathing.

### *Benefits*
• Clears nasal passages.
• Energizes the body.

## ALTERNATE NOSTRIL BREATHING (*NADI SUDHI PRANAYAMA*)

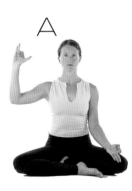

1. Sit comfortably with your spine straight, shoulders relaxed, and chin parallel to the floor.

2. Make a loose fist with your right hand. Release the last two fingers and the thumb, making a V-shape with your hand (Photo A).

3. Take a Deep Three-Part inhalation, expanding through your lower abdomen, then your rib cage, then your upper chest.

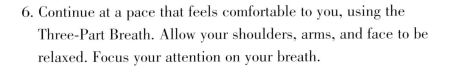

4. Cover your right nostril with your thumb and exhale slowly through your left nostril (Photo B).

5. Inhale through your left nostril, cover your left nostril with your fingers, and exhale through your right nostril.

6. Continue at a pace that feels comfortable to you, using the Three-Part Breath. Allow your shoulders, arms, and face to be relaxed. Focus your attention on your breath.

7. Once the pattern of "exhale, inhale, switch nostril" feels natural, begin to extend your exhalations so that they are longer than your inhalations. Gradually work up to making your exhalations twice as long as your inhalations without straining. A typical round of Alternate Nostril Breathing is 3–5 minutes.

### *Modifications*
• If you are congested, simply stop and go back to doing Deep Three-Part Breathing.

### *Benefits*
• Clears and focuses the mind, especially preceding meditation.
• Triggers a relaxation response in your body.
• Balances both cerebral hemispheres so that logic and intuition may work in harmony in your consciousness.

# CHAPTER THREE

# Creating Your Practice

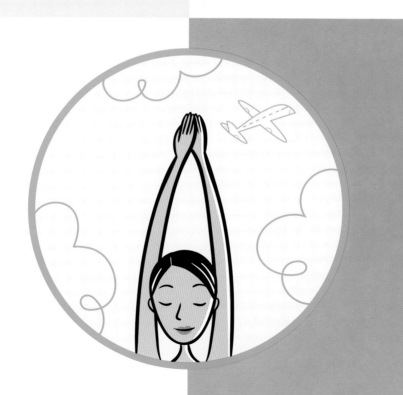

The Hatha yogi should live in a secluded hut free of stones, fire, and dampness to a distance of four cubits in a country that is properly governed, virtuous, prosperous, and peaceful.

—Svatmarama (*The Hatha Yoga Pradipika*, trans. Brian Dana Akers, YogaVidya.com)

Unless your mode of transportation is walking, then traveling involves constricting your body into tight spaces for long periods of time. *Asana* practice decompresses your spine and allows your body to expand back to its rightful, radiant state. Your practice also reconstructs your breath from its restricted, shallow form to a deep, flowing, and steady breath that occurs when you expand in all directions.

## YOUR HOTEL ROOM/YOGA STUDIO

Many hotels around the world carry yoga instructional tapes for their guests to use. Some hotel fitness centers offer drop-in gym classes. But if your hotel or motel does not provide any of these services, you can still make your hotel room yoga-friendly. Hotel and motel rooms, because of their sparseness, make excellent practice spaces. The lack of personal reference can actually aid your efforts to let go of your outer self and tune in deeper to your innermost self.

While yoga is ultimately about going beyond your body, you can still use some items to help you relax your mind and senses. Scented candles or incense used only during practice can induce an automatic relaxation response in your body and mind. There are many safe and portable travel candles available on the market. If you don't have candles or incense, you can dab some lavender oil on your temples and other pressure points. (To wake up, you may want to try peppermint oil instead.) Soft and meditative music can also have the same effect. If you prefer silence, many travel yogis swear by earplugs to drown out noise in hotels, airports, airplanes, cars, and trains.

To practice yoga, wear loose, comfortable clothing. Do not wear shoes or socks. Try to practice on an empty stomach. A sticky mat (available at most sporting good stores and yoga centers) helps keep you from slipping, but you don't really need one as long as you practice on a flat surface. As the routines in this book indicate, you don't even need a conventional exercise space at all.

## HOW TO START AND END A SESSION

Start each session with a few minutes in Simple Sitting Pose (*Sukhasana;* see pages 32–33). Sit comfortably in a cross-legged position. Close your eyes and simply observe the sensations in your body and the thoughts that arise in your mind. Allow your forehead and jaw to relax. Roll your shoulders slowly to release any tension. Allow your shoulder blades to gently press into your back so that your chest opens and your heart lifts.

You may wish to dedicate your practice session to someone at home, or to your True Nature, or to some other being or person outside of yourself. When you feel quiet and centered, continue with your session.

A typical ending sequence to your practice session is to be in Corpse Pose (*Savasana*; see pages 98–99) for 2–5 minutes. If there's time, you can rest in Yogic Sleep (*Yoga Nidra*; see pages 100–104) before Corpse Pose. After Corpse Pose, come back into Simple Sitting Pose (*Sukhasana*) again for whatever breathing exercise (*pranayama*; see pages 104–107) you choose to do.

## OM

Many yogis begin and end their session with three rounds of "OM." OM is a fundamental and untranslatable Sanskrit syllable. It is the traditional chant to center your mind and body before meditation or hatha practice. OM doesn't "mean" anything. It's the basic sound a body makes when the mouth opens and then closes, but the experience of chanting "OM" creates peaceful vibrations in your body and mind. It also releases tension in your throat and directs the flow of energy outward, which is a prelude to what happens on a physical level during *asana* practice. If chanted on a regular basis before and after each yoga session, the sound can also be a mental trigger for relaxation. As you chant, feel the sound vibrating through your solar plexus and head cavity.

Ending a session with "OM" can be an experience of letting go, sending your positive energy out into the world with the knowledge that when you practice you're practicing not just for yourself, but for the people around you.

## YOGA MUDRA

Another tradition in yoga is to end a session with Yoga Mudra (or "Yogic Seal"). A *mudra* is a gesture you make to induce a deeper state of awareness and to augment the life energy in your body. Yoga

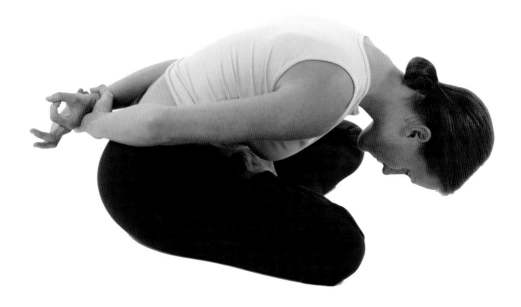

Mudra also prompts release and surrender, signaling the end of your outer work of *asana* and the beginning of your inner work of deep relaxation and meditation. You can do Yoga Mudra before deep relaxation, after OM, or at any point that feels right to you.

Come into Yoga Mudra by sitting comfortably in a cross-legged position. Bring your hands behind your back. Gently hold your right wrist with your left hand. Inhale as you sit up tall. As you exhale, fold forward from your hips with a flat back until your upper body releases down effortlessly toward the floor. Relax for about 30 seconds. Allow your mind to quiet down and your awareness to gather inside. Then, with a flat back, slowly come back up at a pace that suggests the rising of the sun in the morning or the lifting of fog.

# THE MORNING ENERGIZER (20 MINUTES)

*Routine*

• **Sun Breaths (6 times)**
• **Sun Salutation (6 times)**
• **Warrior I (30–45 seconds each side)**
• **Warrior II (30–45 seconds each side)**
• **Triangle Pose (30 seconds each side)**
• **Half Spinal Twist (30–60 seconds each side)**
• **Corpse Pose (5 minutes)**

Early morning is one of the best times of the day to practice hatha yoga. Your mind has yet to become entrenched in its usual grooves and your body is generally at its most relaxed.

Energizing the body-mind through *asana* practice depends on two things: deep inhalations coupled with postures that open your upper and front body and stretch your upper spine. Standing postures and backward bends are ideal for waking up your spine and entire being.

This morning energizer will get your life-force moving while leaving your mind clear and centered.

## SUN BREATHS

1. Stand with your legs about shoulder-width apart. Center your body over your feet with your tailbone pointing down toward the floor, your pelvis centered, and the crown of your head reaching toward the sky.

2. As you inhale deeply, extend your arms out to the sides with palms facing up and then lift your arms up alongside your ears with palms facing each

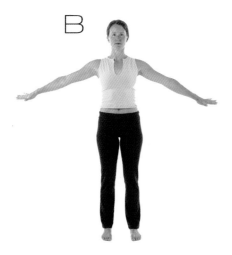

other (Photo A). Keep your shoulder blades moving down your back rather than hunched up toward your ears.

3. On your exhalation, allow your arms to extend out to the sides with palms facing down and then release your arms alongside your body with palms facing in (Photo B). Engage the back of your throat and open your mouth as you exhale. Let your breath escape as a "haaaa" sound.

4. Repeat five times. Imagine that your breath is moving you, always inhaling as you lift your arms, exhaling ("haaaa") as you release your arms down. Take a moment to notice the energy rising up through your body.

## SUN SALUTATION (*SURYA NAMASKAR*)

**Refer to pages 42–48 for the details of each position in Sun Salutation.**

5. Perform Position One: Mountain Pose (*Tadasana;* Photo C).

6. Position Two: Arms Up (Photo D).

7. Position Three: Forward Bend (*Uttanasana;* Photos E, F, and G).

8. Position Four: Lunge (Photo H).

9. Position Five: Downward Facing Dog (Photo I).

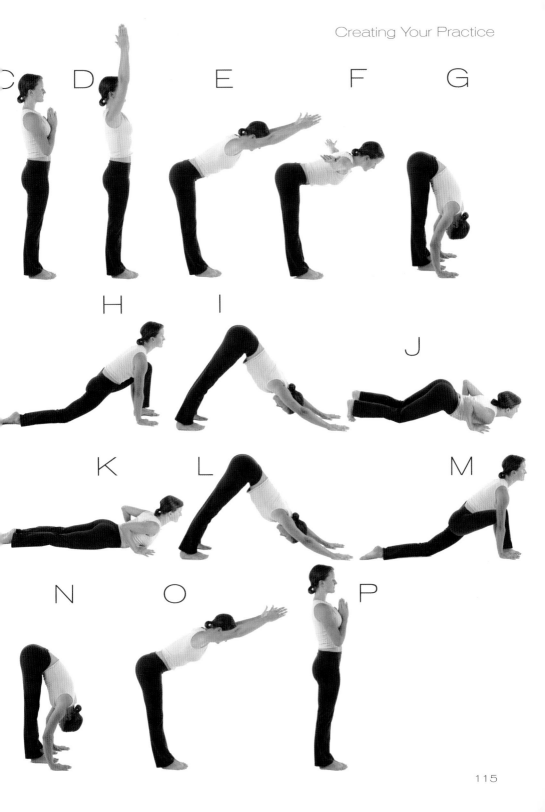

10. Position Six: Knees, Chest, Chin (Photo J).

11. Position Seven: Cobra (Photo K).

12. Position Eight: Downward Facing Dog (Photo L).

13. Position Nine: Lunge (Photo M).

14. Position Ten: Forward Bend (*Uttanasana;* Photo N).

15. Position Eleven: Reverse Dive (Photo O).

16. Position Twelve: Mountain Pose (*Tadasana;* Photo P).

17. Repeat five times, gradually picking up the pace until your body warms up. Stop or slow down if you are short of breath or dizzy. On the final round, instead of swan diving to a forward bend, try rolling down to a standing forward bend. Just hang for a moment and then roll slowly back up, allowing the movement to create space between each vertebra. Pause and notice how you feel.

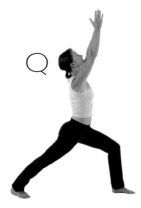

## WARRIOR I (*VIRABHADRASANA I*)
**Refer to pages 82–84 for the details in doing this pose.**
18. Take a wide stand and hold Warrior I (Photo Q) for 30–45 seconds on each side.

## WARRIOR II (*VIRABHADRASANA II*)
**Refer to pages 84–85 for the details in doing this pose.**
19. Open into Warrior II and hold for 30–45 seconds on each side (Photo R). Find your breath and

focus on it while allowing your spine to lengthen. Find and emphasize the back-bending aspect of the posture.

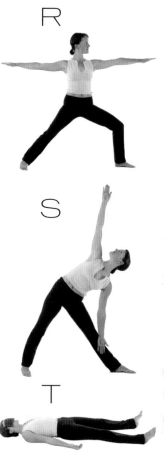

## TRIANGLE (*TRIKONASANA*)

**Refer to pages 86–87 for the details in doing this pose.**

20. Straighten your front leg and slide into Triangle Pose (Photo S). Hold for 30 seconds on each side. Allow your chest to open, creating a surge of energy in your heart center.

## CORPSE POSE (*SAVASANA*)

**Refer to pages 98–99 for the details in doing this pose.**

21. Lie in Corpse Pose for a few breaths (Photo T). You can use an eye pillow while you rest.

## HALF SPINAL TWIST (*ARDHA MATSYENDRASANA*)

**Refer to pages 96–97 for the details in doing this pose.**

22. Sit up with your legs extended out in front of you. Do a Half Spinal Twist for each side (Photo U). Hold about 45 seconds.

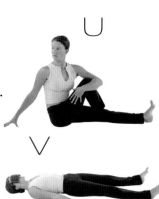

## CORPSE POSE (*SAVASANA*)

**Refer to pages 98–99 for the details in doing this pose.**

23. Lie down in Corpse Pose again (Photo V). This time, rest for 5 minutes. Relax your body, but keep your mind alert and focused on your breath. Visualize how you'd like the rest of your day to unfold.

## THE AFTERNOON DE-STRESSER (20 MINUTES)

*Routine*

- **Simple Sitting Pose (1 minute)**
- **Deep Three-Part Breath (1 minute)**
- **Alternate Nostril Breathing (1 minute)**
- **Diamond Pose (30 seconds)**
- **Child's Pose (a few minutes)**
- **Sun Salutation (2 times)**
- **Corpse Pose (2–3 minutes)**
- **Staff Pose (transitional)**
- **Head-to-Knee Pose (45 seconds each side)**
- **Full Forward Bend (1 minute)**
- **Spinal Twist (20 seconds each side)**
- **Legs Up the Wall (2–3 minutes)**
- **Supported Corpse Pose**

This is a brief routine that will soothe and restore you after a day of sales calls, meetings with demanding clients, or sight-seeing. The most restorative yoga tools are the forward bends and the deep, conscious breathing exercises.

### SIMPLE SITTING POSE (*SUKHASANA*)

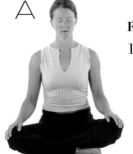

A

**Refer to pages 32–33 for the details in doing this pose.**

1. Settle into a Simple Sitting Pose (Photo A). Center and focus your mind on your breath for a minute.

## DEEP THREE-PART BREATH (*DIRGA SWASAM PRANAYAMA*) AND ALTERNATE NOSTRIL BREATHING (*NADI SUDHI PRANAYAMA*)

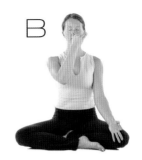

**Refer to pages 104–105 for the detailed steps in Deep Three-Part Breath and pages 106–107 for Alternate Nostril Breathing.**

2. Slowly begin doing your Deep Three-Part Breath for a minute, then ease into Alternate Nostril Breathing (Photo B) for a minute. Sit for a moment feeling the effects of these breathing exercises.

## DIAMOND POSE (*VAJRASANA*) AND CHILD'S POSE (*BALASANA*)

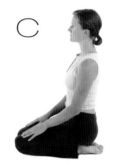

**Refer to page 34 for the detailed steps in Diamond Pose and pages 74–75 for Child's Pose.**

3. Sit back on your heels into Diamond Pose (Photo C). Then fold at your hips and lower your forehead to the floor, surrendering into Child's Pose (Photo D). Release your lower, middle, and upper back, and neck. Feel your blood flowing toward your brain, refreshing your mind. Stay here for at least a minute with your awareness on your breath.

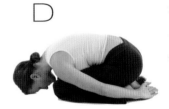

## SUN SALUTATION (*SURYA NAMASKAR*)

**Refer to pages 42–48 for the details of each position in Sun Salutation.**

4. Move slowly through each of the positions, beginning with a mindful Mountain Pose (*Tadasana;* Photo E).

5.  Position Two: Arms Up (Photo F).

6.  Position Three: Forward Bend (*Uttanasana;* Photos G, H, and I).

7.  Position Four: Lunge (Photo J).

8.  Position Five: Downward Facing Dog (Photo K).

9.  Position Six: Knees, Chest, Chin (Photo L).

10. Position Seven: Cobra (Photo M).

11. Position Eight: Downward Facing Dog (Photo N).

12. Position Nine: Lunge (Photo O).

13. Position Ten: Forward Bend (*Uttanasana;* Photo P).

14. Position Eleven: Reverse Dive (Photo Q).

15. Position Twelve: Mountain Pose (*Tadasana;* Photo R).

16. Do another slow round of Sun Salutation.

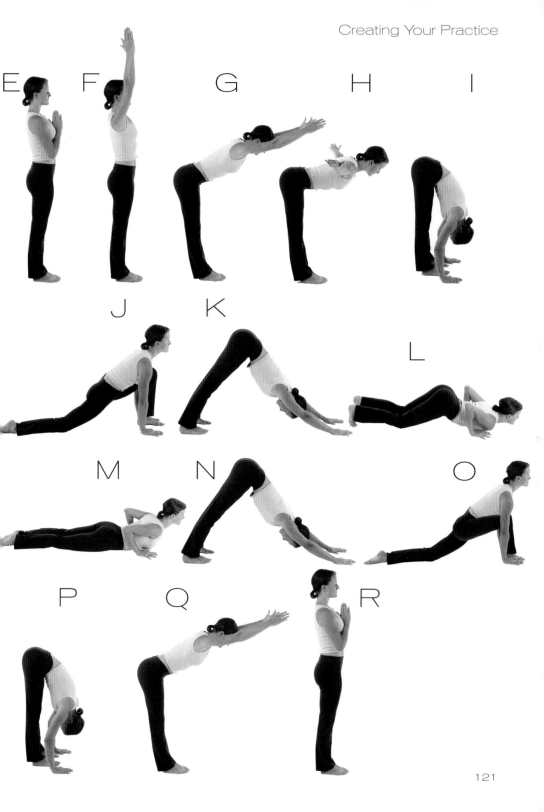

E  F  G  H  I

J  K  L

M  N  O

P  Q  R

## CORPSE POSE (SAVASANA)

**Refer to pages 98–99 for the details in doing this pose.**

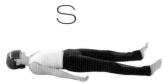

S

17. Lie in Corpse Pose (Photo S) for 2–3 minutes, watching your breath. You can use an eye pillow to relieve eyestrain. If your lower back hurts, allow your shoulder blades to be flat, press your sacrum into the floor, and hug your knees into your chest. Roll from side to side, making circular movements with your knees to massage your lower back.

## THE STAFF POSE (DANDASANA)

**Refer to pages 63–64 for the details in doing this pose.**

T

18. Extend your arms along the floor behind your head and lock your thumbs. Using your abdominal muscles, roll up to a seated posture with your legs extended out in front of your body.

19. Come into Staff Pose (*Dandasana;* Photo T). Make sure to sit at the top of your sitting bones. Rotate your pelvis forward. If your hamstrings are tight, bend your knees slightly but continue to keep your legs activated with your toes pointing up toward the ceiling.

## HEAD-TO-KNEE POSE (JANUSIRSHASANA)

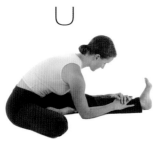

U

**Refer to pages 65–67 for the details in doing this pose.**

20. Draw your right knee in toward your chest while lifting your spine even straighter. Then

open out your right knee to the right side.
Come into Head-to-Knee Pose
(*Janusirshasana;* Photo U). Hold for 45
seconds. Repeat on the other side.

## FULL FORWARD BEND
## (*PASCHIMOTANASANA*)

**Refer to pages 68–69 for the details in doing this pose.**

21. Come back into Staff Pose (*Dandasana;*
    Photo T). Sit up even taller.

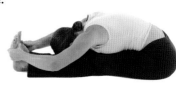

V

22. Rotate your pelvis forward and come
    into Full Forward Bend (*Paschimotanasana;*
    Photo V). Stay in this pose for at least a
    minute. You can place a pillow under your
    forehead for extra comfort.

W

## SIMPLE SITTING POSE
## (*SUKHASANA*)

**Refer to pages 32–33 for the details in doing this pose.**

23. Raise your head and come into a comfortable
    Simple Sitting Pose (Photo W). Twist easily to
    the right, then left. Hold each side for 20 seconds.

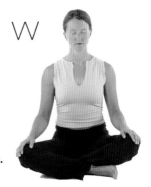

X

## LEGS UP THE WALL
## (*VIPARITA KARANI*)

**Refer to page 81 for the details in doing this pose.**

24. Find an empty wall space and bring yourself
    into Legs Up the Wall (Photo X). Stay in this
    pose for 2–3 minutes.

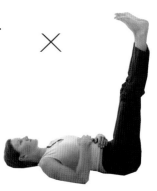

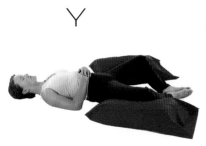

Y

## SUPPORTED CORPSE POSE

25. Finally, lie on your back with the soles of your feet together and your knees out to the side. Use pillows or rolled-up towels under your knees for extra support (Photo Y). Stay in this position until it's time to get up for dinner.

## A GOOD NIGHT'S SLEEP (30 MINUTES)

*Routine*

- **Simple Sitting Pose (1 minute)**
- **Deep Three-Part Breath (2–3 minutes)**
- **Alternate Nostril Breathing (3 minutes)**
- **Cat-Cow (4 times)**
- **Extended Child's Pose (30 seconds)**
- **Downward Facing Dog (30–45 seconds)**
- **Forward Bend (1 minute)**
- **Sun Salutation (1 round)**
- **Corpse Pose (3 minutes)**
- **Cobra (10–15 seconds)**
- **Extended Child's Pose (30 seconds)**
- **Full Forward Bend (45 seconds–1 minute)**
- **Corpse Pose (a few seconds)**
- **Supine Spinal Twist (15 seconds each side)**
- **Corpse Pose (3 minutes)**
- **Yogic Sleep**

The constant stimulation of new sights and sounds, and the basic stress of not being home, can leave your brain constantly "on." A restful practice session before bed can help your brain quiet down for sleep.

# SIMPLE SITTING POSE (SUKHASANA)

**Refer to pages 32–33 for the details in doing this pose.**

1. If you have time, take a soothing, warm shower or bath. Then make yourself some herbal tea. Relax into a Simple Sitting Pose (*Sukhasana;* Photo A) as you sip your tea. Close your eyes and feel the tea's warm vapors rise up to your face. Follow the ins and outs of your breath with your mind, gradually allowing the cares and thoughts of the day to dissolve into complete attention on the present moment.

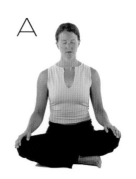

# DEEP THREE-PART BREATH (DIRGA SWASAM PRANAYAMA) AND ALTERNATE NOSTRIL BREATHING (NADI SUDHI PRANAYAMA)

**Refer to pages 104–105 for the detailed steps in Deep Three-Part Breath and pages 106–107 for Alternate Nostril Breathing.**

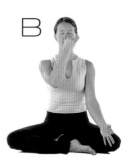

2. Practice Deep Three-Part Breath (*Dirga Swasam Pranayama*) for 2-3 minutes, followed by Alternate Nostril Breathing (*Nadi Sudhi Pranayama;* Photo B) for 3 minutes.

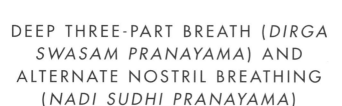

# CAT-COW

**Refer to pages 40–41 for the details in doing this pose.**

3. Gently bring yourself onto your hands and knees for Cat-Cow (Photos C and D). Allow your breath to move your body for at least four repetitions. Keep your awareness on your breath.

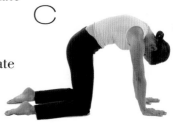

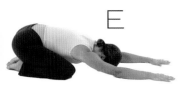

## EXTENDED CHILD'S POSE

**Refer to page 75 for the details in doing this pose.**

4. Stretch into Extended Child's Pose (Photo E). Breathe slowly and rhythmically for about 30 seconds.

## DOWNWARD FACING DOG

**Refer to page 45 for the details in doing this pose.**

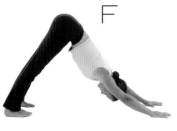

5. Curl your toes under; lift your hips up toward the ceiling and back toward the wall behind you. Come up onto your toes, lift your pelvis, and let your heels sink back to the floor as you come into Downward Facing Dog (Photo F). Breathe deeply, slowly, and hold the posture for 30–45 seconds.

## FORWARD BEND (*UTTANASANA*)

**Refer to page 44 for the details in doing this pose.**

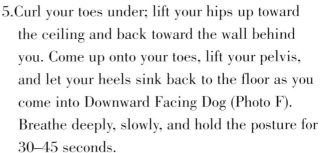

6. Bend your knees and walk slowly toward your hands as you come into a Forward Bend (Photo G). Allow your spine to lengthen; feel the blood flowing to your brain. Hang for about a minute or as long as you feel comfortable. Bend your knees, tuck your chin, and slowly roll back up to standing.

## SUN SALUTATION (*SURYA NAMASKAR*)

**Refer to pages 42–48 for the details of each position in Sun Salutation.**

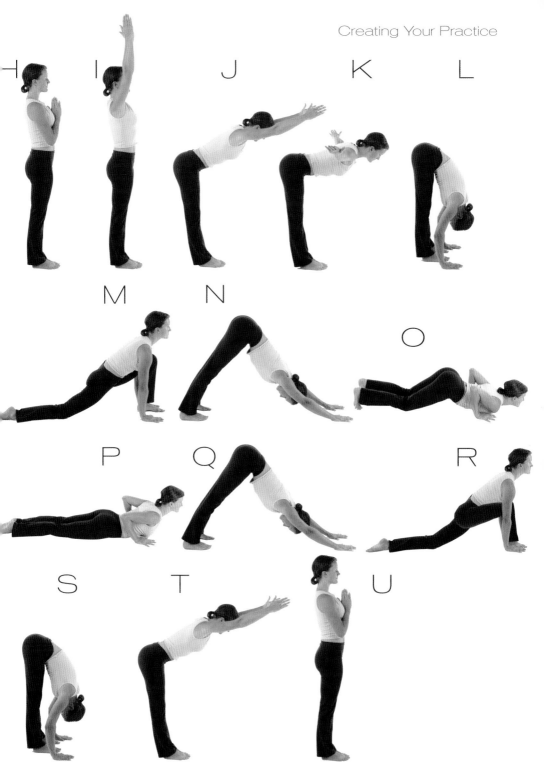

7. Move slowly through each of the positions in your Sun Salutation, beginning with a mindful Mountain Pose (*Tadasana*; Photo H).

8. Position Two: Arms Up (Photo I).

9. Position Three: Forward Bend (*Uttanasana*; Photos J, K, and L).

10. Position Four: Lunge (Photo M).

11. Position Five: Downward Facing Dog (Photo N).

12. Position Six: Knees, Chest, Chin (Photo O).

13. Position Seven: Cobra (Photo P).

14. Position Eight: Downward Facing Dog (Photo Q).

15. Position Nine: Lunge (Photo R).

16. Position Ten: Forward Bend (*Uttanasana*; Photo S).

17. Position Eleven: Reverse Dive (Photo T).

18. Position Twelve: Mountain Pose (*Tadasana*; Photo U).

## CORPSE POSE (SAVASANA)

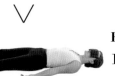

**Refer to pages 98–99 for the details in doing this pose.**

19. Lie down on the floor and rest in Corpse Pose (Photo V) for 3 minutes. You can use an eye pillow while you rest. Observe your breath.

## THE COBRA (*BHUJANGASANA*)

**Refer to pages 49–50 for the details in doing this pose.**

20. Roll over onto your abdomen and relax completely for 30 seconds. Place your palms on the floor underneath your shoulders. Lengthen and release into the Cobra (Photo W). As you inhale, continue to lengthen and release for 10–15 seconds, then slowly lower down. Keep your hands in place, turn your cheek to the side, and relax the legs for a few breaths. Then do another round of Cobra.

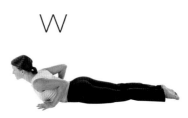

## EXTENDED CHILD'S POSE

**Refer to page 75 for the details in doing this pose.**

21. With your hands still positioned under your shoulders, push yourself back onto all fours. Then sit back on your heels and stretch forward into Extended Child's Pose (Photo X). Hold for 30 seconds or as long as is comfortable for you. Breathe into your lower back.

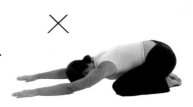

## FULL FORWARD BEND (*PASCHIMOTANASANA*)

**Refer to pages 68–69 for the details in doing this pose.**

22. Tuck your chin into your chest and sit back on your heels. Roll slowly, vertebra by vertebra, into a sitting position. Release your buttocks to the side and extend the legs straight in front of you for a Full Forward Bend (Photo Y). Hold for 45 seconds to 1 minute.

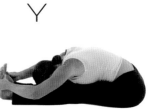

## CORPSE POSE (*SAVASANA*)

**Refer to pages 98–99 for the details in doing this pose.**

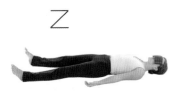

23. Extend your arms alongside your ears and rise up with a flat back, or simply sit slowly back up while walking your hands toward your trunk. Then roll down into Corpse Pose (Photo Z). Relax your body for a few breaths. You can use an eye pillow while you rest.

## SUPINE SPINAL TWIST (*JATHARA PARIVARTANASANA*)

**Refer to pages 94–95 for the details in doing this pose.**

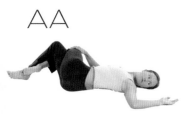

24. Draw your knees into your chest and extend your arms out to the sides at shoulder height. Lower your knees to the right as you bring your left ear to the ground (Photo AA). Loosen your entire body. Hold for 15 seconds. Then do the other side.

## CORPSE POSE AND YOGIC SLEEP

**Refer to pages 98–99 for Corpse Pose and pages 100–104 for Yogic Sleep.**

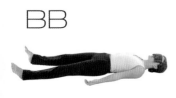

25. Release your head, hands, and legs into Corpse Pose. Lay in Corpse Pose (Photo BB) for about 3 minutes and then transition into Yogic Sleep. An eye pillow can help you settle deeper into your relaxation.

## AIRPLANE YOGA

### *Before You Fly*

If you have time before your flight, find a place to sit down (a chair is always nice, but your carry-on bag or even the floor will do in a pinch).

## SIMPLE SITTING POSE (*SUKHASANA*)

**Refer to pages 32–33 for the details in doing this pose.**

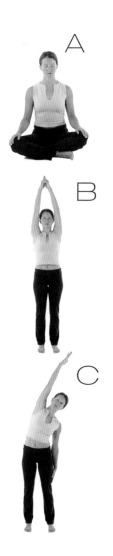

1. If there's room, sit in a Simple Sitting Pose (Photo A). If not, sit on your chair or luggage with your feet flat on the floor and hands resting, palms up, on your knees or thighs. Take a moment to actively notice your surroundings: colors, sounds, smells. Then close your eyes, take a deep breath, and focus on your internal "view": your sensations, breath, emotions, and thoughts. You don't need to block out sounds you may hear, or the occasional disturbances. Just take note of them and let your attention go back within.

## CRESCENT MOON (*ARDHA CHANDRASANA*)

2. Right before you board, stand up. Inhale and stretch your arms up alongside your ears. Interlace your fingers. Point your index fingers toward the ceiling (Photo B). Exhale.

3. On your next inhalation, elongate up. As you exhale, arch over to the left, lengthening the right side of your body while keeping the left side of your body as long and extended as possible (Photo C). Hold for a breath, and then come back to center.

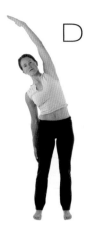

D

4. Inhale and lift your spine. Exhale and arch over to the right (Photo D). Continue this pattern twice more on each side. Be sure to keep your body long rather than bending at the waist.

### Preflight Jitters (or "Flying Anxiety")

Fear of flying is a common and rational response to the unnatural experience of sitting in an airtight box suspended miles above the earth. Deep Three-Part Breath (*Dirga Swasam*; see pages 104–105) can help at any point in your flight. It triggers a relaxation response and introduces more oxygen to the body, thus clearing the mind of cluttered thoughts that may complicate your fear.

Another wonderful yogic tool is Yogic Sleep (*Yoga Nidra*; see pages 100–104). As soon as you are settled into your seat (and after the steward's safety instructions demonstration), begin a seated Yogic Sleep by progressively tuning into and relaxing each major part of your body. You may want to record the instructions for Yogic Sleep onto a cassette and play it back on your Walkman so you can follow along at a soothing pace. When your body is completely relaxed, and your mind is open and responsive, allow some affirmations of trust and courage to penetrate your consciousness:

"I am completely relaxed."

"I ride the waves of life with pleasure and openness."

"I allow fear to transform into exhilaration."

While your mind is receptive, you may want to visualize positive outcomes for your trip ahead. Tell yourself that your business trip will have a smooth and fair result, or that your vacation will be fun and safe.

While the physical practices of yoga can provide comfort, it's the philosophy of yoga that ultimately provides strength in times of fear.

In the yogic philosophy, you *have* a body and a mind, but you don't identify with them as your true self. Your fears are predicated on the belief that you *are* your body and mind—the least enduring aspects of your being.

When you start to identify with your true self that is indestructible and eternal, then your fears will begin to recede. (See also "Anxiety," page 198.)

### *Clearing the Ears*

Many people experience pressure in their ears during lift-off or landing. To clear the ears, and to dissolve facial tension, perform a modified Lion Pose (*Simhasana*; see page 39) in your seat.

1. Take a comfortable inhalation through your nose.

2. As you exhale, open your eyes wide; open your mouth and stick your tongue way down toward your chin. Do this a few times during lift-off and repeat when the plane starts its descent. If you're feeling uninhibited, you can let out a little "roar" to release tension in your throat.

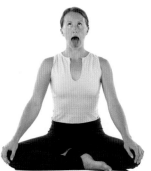

### *Mile-High Yoga*

Whether you're in business class or coach, sitting still for an extended period of time can wreak havoc on your back and body's circulation. In addition, the lack of movement in an already oxygen-depleted atmosphere can cause light-headedness and fatigue.

Unless your goal is to sleep on the flight (see "Jet Lag," page 194), it's important to stay attentive and active.

### *Posture and Awareness*

The first yogic move you can make is to sit deliberately—alert and tall—rather than to slump in your seat. Good posture encourages deeper breathing, good digestion, and an open flow of vital energy to your limbs and organs. Poor posture makes your heart work harder, compresses your colon and other internal organs, and cuts off circulation.

To sit properly, first imagine a string at the top of your cranium, pulling your head up toward the ceiling and lengthening your neck gracefully. Gently press the sitting bones of your buttocks back and away into the seat. Softly engage your abdomen and use your back's strength to stay upright. Use the airline's pillow, a rolled-up towel, or T-shirt as a lumbar support by slipping it into the space between the back of the seat and your lower spine.

Next, pay attention to your feet. Spread your toes and wiggle them around. Consciously allow your feet to be open and broad rather than scrunched up in your shoes.

### *In-flight Stretches*

About 20 minutes into your flight, engage in these conscious stretches.

1. Inhale deeply as you raise your arms up alongside your ears. Bend your elbows and grab hold of opposite elbows (Photo A). Lengthen your torso up and up. . . . Bring your arms a little further back and lift your chest, gently opening your heart. Breathe deeply.

2. With your torso long, exhale and twist easily to the right (Photo B). Hold for a breath, then exhale as you twist easily to the left without straining. Relax your arms down by your sides.

3. Inhale your shoulders up to ears; exhale as you circle your shoulders back and down. Repeat, using your breath to move your shoulders.

4. Grab hold of opposite elbows and lift your arms so they're perpendicular to your chest (à la *I Dream of Jeannie*). Keeping the arms parallel to the floor, drop your head forward, tucking your chin under (Photo C). Hold for a few breaths, allowing the back of your neck to stretch.

5. Carefully allow your left ear to come over your left shoulder. Hold for a few breaths. Then allow your right ear to come down over your right shoulder. Hold for a few breaths. With the next inhalation, feel the head lifting back up. Repeat these stretches every hour that you are onboard, bringing a focused awareness to every breath and movement.

### *Eyestrain*

Tension headaches can crop up when you keep your eyes focused on one thing for too long (see also "Yoga Routines for Common Travel Ailments," page 145). Give your eyes a break by doing these few eye exercises:

1. Gaze at the headrest in front of you for a breath, then shift your focus several feet in front of you for a breath. Repeat five to ten times, letting your eyes move easily without strain.

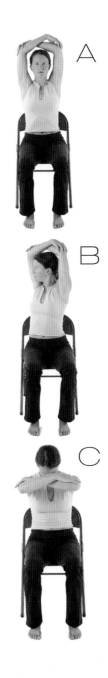

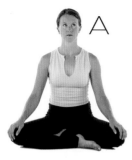

2. Follow this up with slow, easy eye circles according to the Eye Movements (*Netra Vyaayaamam*; see page 35) sequence (Photos A and B). Roll your eyes in both directions—clockwise and counterclockwise. Allow your eyes to seek the periphery of your vision to release fatigue and pressure in your optic muscles.

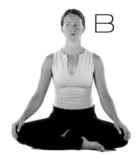

### Walking "On Air" Meditation

At least once during your plane trip, get up and take a mindful stroll to the restroom. Stand tall; notice the feeling of your feet on the floor. Notice the sounds, smells, and colors inside the plane. When you reach the bathroom, shake out your arms and legs, releasing any tightness.

### After Landing

After subjecting your hips to tiny airplane seats, they cry out for some opening. Following your arrival (perhaps while waiting at the baggage carousel or a rest area), find a place to sit in a modified Bound Angle (*Baddha Konasana*; see pages 72–73).

1. Bring the soles of your feet together with the knees relaxed out to the sides. Hold onto your ankles (Photo A). Move your shoulder blades down your back. Lift your chest.

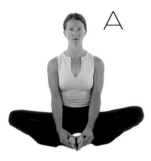

2. Engage in a Deep Three-Part Breath (*Dirga Swasam*; see pages 104–105). Hold this position for at least 30 seconds.

## STARFISH

3. If you can't find a place to sit, simply assume a wide-leg stance and open your arms with your palms facing forward. Widen your fingers, face, and feet (Photo B). Pretend you are a starfish and stretch out in all directions.

### *Jet Lag*

Jet lag is fatigue brought on by poor air quality in planes and the body's attempt to adjust rapidly to a new time zone. Jet lag, like any other stress-related symptom in the body, can be prevented or at least diminished with diet, listening to your body, and conscious breathing.

Not every traveler experiences jet lag. Many are able to fly through different time zones with no ill effects. Your thoughts are powerful. A quietly confident expectancy of good health can have a positive influence on how you feel.

As soon as you board the plane, set your watch to your destination time and act as if it were that time. Stay hydrated by drinking lots of water and avoid beverages like coffee and alcohol. (See Chapter Four for more advice about how to eat on the road and in the air.) Breathe deeply whenever you can remember to and keep your body moving (see "Walking 'On Air' Meditation," page 136) if it is daytime at your destination.

When you get to your destination, try to stay awake until it's actually bedtime in that location. Do the "Morning Energizer" routine (see pages 113–117) or engage in some activity—conscious exercise or brisk walking—to invigorate your body and mind.

## CAR YOGA

The conditions of driving are similar to those of flying: small seats and not much room for movement. The advantage, of course, is that as a driver (or assertive passenger) you can control your itinerary by making stops along the way.

### *Posture and Awareness*

As with "Airplane Yoga," you can overcome the effects of being wedged into tight spaces by sitting properly without slouching. Press your sitting bones deliberately down into your seat to allow your spine to be long. Contract your abdomen slightly and keep your shoulders rotated back and down. Bring a pillow or rolled-up towel to support your lumbar spine.

### *Stretch Breaks*

The rule of thumb for long-distance road trips is to stop every 2 hours (or every 100 miles) for a good stretch. Try these simple but effective stretches.

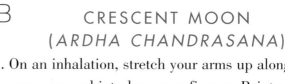

A    B

## CRESCENT MOON (*ARDHA CHANDRASANA*)

1. On an inhalation, stretch your arms up alongside your ears and interlace your fingers. Point your index fingers toward the ceiling (Photo A).

2. On your next inhalation, elongate up. As you exhale, arch over to the left, lengthening the right side of your body while keeping the left side of your body as long and extended as possible (Photo B). Hold for a breath, and then come back to center.

3. Inhale and lift your spine. Exhale and arch over to the right (Photo C). Continue this pattern twice more on each side. Be sure to keep your body long rather than bending at the waist.

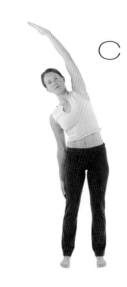

### *Chest Opener*

1. Sit comfortably in your seat with feet about hip distance apart. Interlace your fingers behind your back with your palms facing in. Roll your shoulders back and lightly squeeze your shoulder blades together (Photo A). Inhale, lifting your heart; exhale, stretching your arms back. Hold for three deep, conscious breaths.

2. Inhale deeply. On the exhale, bend your elbows and bring your clasped hands to the right side of your rib cage (Photo B). Hold for a breath and repeat on the left side.

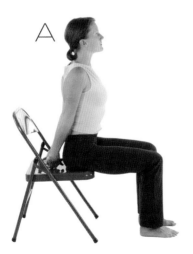

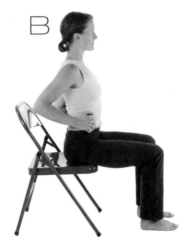

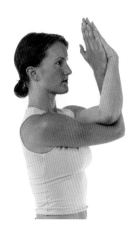

### Back Opener

1. Sit or stand tall with your chest lifted and your tailbone tucked slightly under. Inhale and raise your arms to shoulder height.

2. Exhale and bring your right arm under your left. Bend your elbows and press your palms.

3. Encourage your elbows down toward your navel by bringing your fingertips below the level of your nose. Hold for three breaths and release. Reverse your arms and hold for three more breaths.

### Shoulder Rolls

1. Inhale your shoulders up to your ears.

2. Exhale as you bring your shoulders back and down. Move your shoulder blades deeply down your back. Repeat three times, allowing the breath to guide the movement.

## SEATED STRETCHES

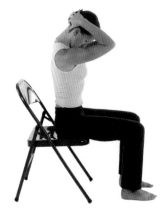

Here are four seated stretches for passengers to do during the car ride—or for drivers only when cars are parked.

### Forward Neck Stretch

1. Interlace your fingers and clasp them behind your head at the base of your skull. Allow your chin to drop down near your chest.

2. Let gravity and the weight of your hands stretch the back of your neck. Hold for three to five deep breaths.

### Side Neck Stretch

1. If you're in a vehicle with bucket seats, sit forward on the seat with your feet planted squarely and firmly on the floor. Reach your right hand back and grasp the right side of the seat. Lengthen your spine; tuck your chin into your chest.

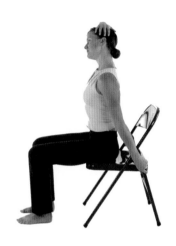

2. Pull your body to the left and place your left hand on the right side of your head. Carefully pull your head toward the left. Hold for three deep breaths and then switch to the other side.

**NOTE:** If your vehicle does not have bucket seats, instead of reaching back to grasp the side of the seat, you can simply leave the non-pulling arm on its respective knee.

### Seated Twist

With your feet squarely on floor, bring your left hand to the outside of your right knee and twist easily to the right. Try looking out over your right shoulder. Hold for three breaths and then reverse the twist with your right hand on your left knee.

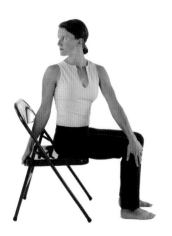

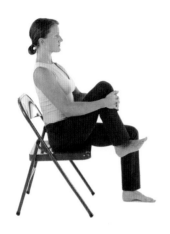

## SEATED LEG STRETCH
### (*PAVANA MUKTASANA*)

1. Sit up straight and tall with your back moving away from the seat.

2. Inhaling, lift your right leg up off the floor and hold your right knee with interlaced hands. Keep your shoulders rolled back and your chest lifted. Continue to pull your knee in closer to your body with every exhalation. Hold for three to five breaths and then repeat on the other leg.

### *Yogic Driving*

If you're the driver on the trip, you have the privilege (and duty) of observing mindful concentration while operating the car. Some people like to drink coffee on long-distance drives in order to stave off sleepiness, but caffeine creates a false and short-lived feeling of energy in the body/mind. Being a "rajasic" or heat-producing food (see pages 187–189), it doesn't promote the peace of mind that we seek in yogic traveling. Instead, begin every segment of driving with some Rapid Diaphragmatic Breathing (*Kapalabhati*; see page 106) to liven up your nervous system and help you stay alert as much as possible.

Another misguided method for staying alert or being entertained on the road is to crank up the radio to a loud volume. The truth is, music—even played at deafening volumes—can become as lulling as white noise once your ears become acclimated to the radio's sounds and rhythm. The volume can also keep you from hearing sounds you may need to hear.

It is far better to sing spiritedly as you drive. Singing aids deeper breathing, which oxygenates your body and keeps your mind lively. It releases endorphins into your bloodstream, promoting cheerfulness. Studies show that it may even boost your immune system. And, of course, it's fun and social, too.

Another way to avoid driving while sleepy is to schedule your drive times so that they don't coincide with the body's natural "downtime." This usually happens in the late afternoon (approximately 3:00 PM) and the early morning (between 2:00 and 4:00 AM).

While you are driving, staring ahead at the pavement can be mesmerizing. So, even as you keep your eyes on the road, allow them to shift and move regularly by sweeping your eyes from one side of the view ahead to the other.

When you arrive at your destination, give your body one last stretch: inhale, sweep your arms up alongside your ears; exhale, lower your arms down. Shake your legs and arms lightly, allowing the circulation to return to your limbs.

You can thank your car for getting you to your destination safely.

## TRAIN YOGA

Train travel takes longer, but there are many benefits to it. It offers slightly roomier accommodations (especially if you go first class) than planes do. The journey occurs at an easier pace and provides beautiful window views. Going by train can also provide you with a sense of groundedness, as you can see the actual accumulation of miles under your wheels. This makes the travel seem less abstract.

The downside of train travel is the possibility of delays. It's common for trains to be late. Sometimes the train comes to a dead stop—maybe for hours—with no explanation from the crew. Further, the sometimes bouncy ride and seeming endlessness of a long trek can wear out your patience.

There are practical considerations that make train travel more comfortable. If you can fit it in with your luggage, bring your own blanket, pillow, and snacks (see Chapter Four). Meanwhile, take advantage of the relative spaciousness of the train by regularly doing some walking meditation (see page 136) up and down the aisles. You can also stretch in the same ways described in the airplane and car yoga sections (see pages 131–143).

## TRAIN *TADASANA*

The lulls and rocking motion of the train can be alternately relaxing and jarring. Practicing Mountain Pose (*Tadasana*) can soothe your mind and deepen your experience. (This posture is fun to do on subways, buses, and short train trips, too.) Like surfing the bumps and waves of life, Train *Tadasana* requires balance and mental poise. This practice is calming, and induces patience and acceptance.

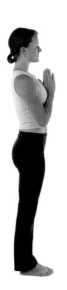

1. Find a place to stand in your compartment (or in a public area on the train) where you won't be blocking anyone. Stand in your best Mountain Pose: shoulders rolled back and down, heart opened and slightly lifting, spine vertical, and legs standing wide apart for balance, if necessary.

2. Imagine extending your energy down through your legs, up through the top of your head, and feel your whole body vibrating with energy and light. If any place in your body feels tense, gently direct your breath there, letting the tension dissolve.

3. Now focus on steadying your breath and bringing your awareness into your body. You don't need to close your eyes, but stay tuned in to the sensations within your body, investigating the symphony of feelings happening there. Feel how your body responds to the movement of the train. See if you can remain completely still and open and watchful, observing the subtle adjustments that your body makes automatically. You can also watch your thoughts come and go in dialogue with the activity around you.

## YOGA ROUTINES FOR COMMON TRAVEL AILMENTS
## HEADACHE

### Tension Headache

Occasional headaches can be caused by any number of things, but the common denominator is tension—particularly in the scalp, neck, and shoulders. People sometimes contract their muscles as an unconscious response to stress. It can also occur while being confined to small spaces without taking the time to consciously move or expand. Muscular tension in this region reduces blood flow to the surrounding areas, causing mild to sharp pain, typically in the temples and at the base of the neck. (If you have chronic or severe headaches, please consult your physician for diagnosis and treatment.)

What you want to avoid when you have a headache are postures (such as excessive forward bends or inversions) that change the pressure in your head. Instead, focus on soothing your nerves with breathing exercises and gently stretching the contracted areas.

### SIMPLE SITTING POSE (SUKHASANA)

**Refer to pages 32–33 for the details in doing this pose.**

1. Settle into a Simple Sitting Pose. Center and focus your mind on your breath.

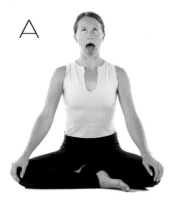

## LION POSE (*SIMHASANA*)

**Refer to page 39 for the details in doing this pose.**

2. Slowly open your eyes and then open your whole face into Lion (Photo A). Quietly "roar."

3. Let your chin fall down easily toward the chest, stretching the back of the neck. (If this makes the pain worse, then allow your head to come back up to center and proceed to step 4, Diamond Pose.) Breathe deeply. On about the fourth inhalation, let your head come back up. Carefully allow your left ear to inch toward your left shoulder. Hold for a few breaths. Repeat on the right side.

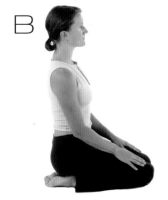

## DIAMOND POSE (*VAJRASANA*)

**Refer to page 34 for the details in doing this pose.**

4. Come into Diamond Pose (Photo B). Reach your arms behind your body, interlacing fingers with your palms together and knuckles facing away. Squeeze the shoulder blades, lifting the heart, breathing consciously for three complete breaths.

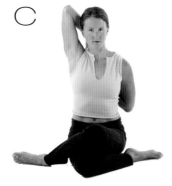

## COW FACE POSE (*GOMUKHASANA*)

**Refer to pages 70–71 for the details in doing this pose.**

5. Raise up your right arm alongside your right ear. Bend your elbow, reaching right fingertips toward your left shoulder blade. Bend your left elbow behind your back and try to touch the

fingertips of both hands together, keeping your chest lifted (Photo C). Breathe into your shoulders for three breaths. Reverse your arms.

## HALF SPINAL TWIST
## (ARDHA MATSYENDRASANA)

**Refer to pages 96–97 for the details in doing this pose.**

6. Allow your hips to fall over to the right and extend your legs out in front of you. Swing your right leg over your left and twist to the right (Photo D). Hold for about 30 seconds. Pay special attention to the sensations in your shoulders. Repeat on the other side.

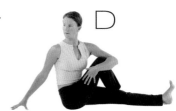

## THE COBRA
## (BHUJANGASANA)

**Refer to pages 49–50 for the details in doing this pose.**

7. Lie on your abdomen and come into Cobra Pose (Photo E). Breathe into your shoulder blades and hold for three deep breaths. Try not to tense your shoulders or neck. Imagine the flow of energy from your navel through your upper body and then through the crown of your head. Repeat.

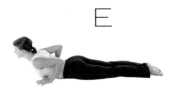

## CORPSE POSE (SAVASANA)

**Refer to pages 98–99 for the details in doing this pose.**

8. Come into Corpse Pose (Photo F) and hold for three breaths. You can use an eye pillow while you rest.

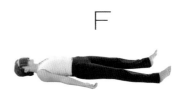

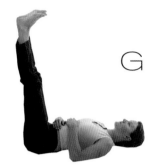

G

## LEGS UP THE WALL (*VIPARITA KARANI*)

**Refer to page 81 for the details in doing this pose.**

9.   Find an available wall space and come into
     Legs Up the Wall (Photo G). Make sure your
     shoulder blades are flat on the floor. Hold for
     3 minutes with an awareness of your breath.

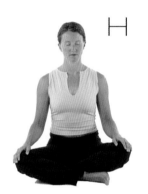

H

## SIMPLE SITTING POSE (*SUKHASANA*) AND ALTERNATE NOSTRIL BREATHING (*NADI SUDHI PRANAYAMA*)

**Refer to pages 32–33 for the detailed steps in Simple
Sitting Pose and pages 106–107 for Alternate Nostril
Breathing.**

10.  Sit in Simple Sitting Pose (*Sukhasana;* Photo
     H) and perform Alternate Nostril Breathing
     (*Nadi Sudhi Pranayama;* Photo I) for about
     3 minutes.

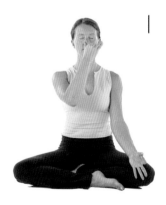

I

## YOGIC SLEEP (*YOGA NIDRA*)

**Refer to pages 100–104 for the details in doing this pose.**

11.  If you have an extra 20 minutes, end your
     session with Yogic Sleep.

### *Eyestrain*

Headaches can occur in the front part of your head
and around your eyes. Prevent eyestrain headaches
by performing this practice daily, but listen to your
body. If doing these movements actually makes
your eyes ache more, then stop.

## EYE MOVEMENTS (*NETRA VYAAYAAMAM*)

**Refer to page 35 for the details in doing this pose.**

1. Mindfully and slowly circle your eyes in a clockwise direction (Photos A and B). Do this several times, then move your eyes in a counterclockwise direction.

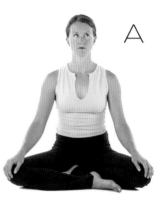

## LION POSE (*SIMHASANA*)

**Refer to page 39 for the details in doing this pose.**

2. Follow with a few rounds of Lion Pose (Photo C) to loosen up your head and scalp.

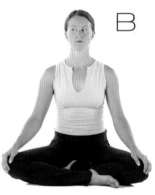

# NAUSEA OR MOTION SICKNESS

The irregular motion of cars, trains, buses, and boats can disturb the vestibular system of your inner ear, which stimulates the vomiting center of your brain. Sometimes motion sickness is set off by conflicting information about motion. For example, your eyes are reading a book, but your inner ear is responding to the bumps and sways of the train, car, or plane.

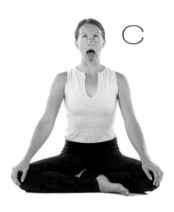

One way to cope with this kind of nausea (or to prevent it from happening) is to limit the amount of information being taken in. You can close your eyes, wear earplugs, or, if in a car, keep your vision on the horizon in order to match the information that the middle ear is receiving. (See also pages 194–195 for nutritional recommendations for preventing motion sickness.)

Doing variations of Deep Three-Part Breath and Alternate Nostril Breathing may also pacify a shaky stomach. Instead of your regular breathing, use Ujjayi (pronounced: oo-jie) breathing during these exercises. Ujjayi breathing is done with your mouth closed and gently tightening the back of your throat. The sound you make should be similar to the roar of the ocean.

## DEEP THREE-PART BREATH
### (*DIRGA SWASAM PRANAYAMA*)

**Refer to pages 104–105 for the details in this exercise.**

1. Sit comfortably and begin your Deep Three-Part Breath. After you have the rhythm down, start your Ujjayi breathing by exhaling with an open mouth. Make a "haaa" sound as if you were blowing on your glasses before cleaning them. Focus on the sound of your breath. Allow the sound and the deep breathing to soothe you. Do this for several minutes.

## ALTERNATE NOSTRIL BREATHING
### (*NADI SUDHI PRANAYAMA*)

**Refer to pages 106–107 for the details in this exercise.**

2. Close your lips and continue with your Ujjayi breathing as you begin Alternate Nostril Breathing. Engage the back of your throat on the exhalations. This will slow down the exhalations considerably, which will calm your nervous system and midbrain.

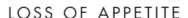

## LOSS OF APPETITE

If travel has disrupted your eating pattern, or if stress has caused your appetite to disappear, then get the digestive fires burning again with this brief routine.

## CORPSE POSE (SAVASANA)

**Refer to pages 98–99 for the details in doing this pose.**

1. Lie on your back and take a few deep, centering breaths (Photo A). You can use an eye pillow while you rest.

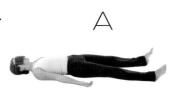

## THE COBRA (BHUJANGASANA)

**Refer to pages 49–50 for the details in doing this pose.**

2. Gently roll over onto your stomach. Take a few more deep breaths, allowing your body to release completely. Then bring your palms to the floor under your shoulders. Lift your chest and head (Photo B). Hold for 15 seconds. Release, then repeat.

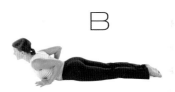

## FULL LOCUST (SALABHASANA)

**Refer to pages 53–54 for the details in doing this pose.**

3. Take a few breaths. Bring your arms under you. Place your chin on the floor and then lift both legs (Photo C). Hold for 30–60 seconds.

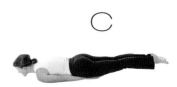

## HALF SPINAL TWIST (ARDHA MATSYENDRASANA)

**Refer to pages 96–97 for the details in doing this pose.**

4. Roll over onto your back. Bend your knees, roll over to your right side, and use your hands to push yourself up into a seated position. Bring your right leg over your left and twist to the right (Photo D). Hold for 30–60 seconds. Repeat on the other side.

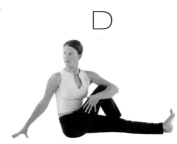

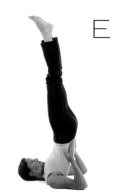

E

## SHOULDER STAND (*SARVANGASANA*)

**Refer to pages 76–78 for the details in doing this pose.**

5. Lie down on your back, bring your arms alongside your body. Swing your legs overhead and then lift them up toward the ceiling (Photo E). Hold for 1–3 minutes. Bring your legs down.

## THE FISH (*MATSYASANA*)

**Refer to pages 58–60 for the details in doing this pose.**

6. With your legs together, move your pelvis toward your feet and lift your rib cage high up into the air. Arch your upper body. Let your head relax back and lower the top of your head to the floor (Photo F). Hold for as long as you feel comfortable. Release and lie in Corpse Pose.

F

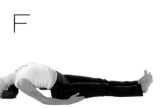

## RAPID DIAPHRAGMATIC BREATHING (*KAPALABHATI*) AND ALTERNATE NOSTRIL BREATHING (*NADI SUDHI*)

**Refer to page 106 for the detailed steps in Rapid Diaphragmatic Breathing and pages 106–107 for Alternate Nostril Breathing.**

7. Bend your knees, roll over to one side, and sit up slowly. Engage in Rapid Diaphragmatic Breathing for a minute and then Alternate Nostril Breathing for up to 2 minutes. Then rest easily for a few minutes.

## ANGER AND FRUSTRATION

Despite having the best intentions and being fully prepared for your trip, you can still experience moments of anger and frustration in response to the stress of travel. These emotions flicker in your mind first as thoughts and then manifest in your body. Through the practice of yoga, you can work toward an awareness of the fluctuations in your mind. If you can catch an angry thought before it turns into a full-body experience, you have taken a giant step toward self-control and embodying the peaceful truth of your being. But sometimes those thoughts still slip through the cracks and turn into ire and despair. Unchecked, they may even grow into "road rage."

### *Stopping, Observing, and Communicating*

When you find yourself becoming angry, the first step you can take is to give yourself a "time out." Even if you can't physically step aside from the stressful situation, you can pause a moment and take three full, deep breaths to clear your mind. These deep breaths are like hitting a "reset" button inside yourself that is often enough to sweep your mind and body clear of hostility.

If not, then the next step in coping with anger is to observe your body's reactions. You can be a scientist or anthropologist of your body simply by observing nonjudgmentally what happens when anger arises: "My throat constricts. My breathing is shallower. I feel a pain between my eyebrows. . . ." By doing this, you anchor yourself in your body for a moment and just feel all the sensations of your emotion, letting it all pass through you without letting it get "stuck" anywhere. With focused and dispassionate attention to the processes of your body, you can often watch your emotions come and go like a passing storm. It's when you resist your emotions, or blindly lash out, that they take on a dark or harmful quality.

The third step is to assess whether communication is possible. For example, if your anger has arisen from a random rudeness by a stranger, it may not be advantageous or even possible to confront that person. But if the opportunity presents itself, and you are calm enough to express your feelings without getting upset, then you can try to express your exasperation in a non-blaming way. This sort of polite honesty can disarm even the most self-absorbed person and nudge them out of the bubble of their own self. A lot of times people aren't aware of their own rudeness and the information comes as a surprise. They may apologize, or they may even explain their behavior in a way that makes you aware of the whole picture. On the other hand, they may react with defensiveness and spite. The response doesn't matter—just the act of expressing yourself can be enough to bring you back to calm.

### *Relaxing and Roaring*

Here are some yoga poses that may help you deal with the energy of anger.

## YOGIC SLEEP (*YOGA NIDRA*)

**Refer to pages 100–104 for the details in doing this pose.**

1. Lie down and clench your entire body in order to squeeze out the tension. Release and make room for blood flow, energy, and relaxation. Do this a few times until you feel calmer.

## LION POSE (*SIMHASANA*)

**Refer to page 39 for the details in doing this pose.**

2. Sit comfortably and do a few spirited rounds of Lion. Letting out some loud growls will provide a great release for animosity and frustration.

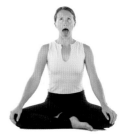

# CONSTIPATION

When you sit for long periods of time in cramped conditions, you run the risk of compressing your colon and causing constipation. A good sitting posture is usually enough to counterbalance this. Gently lengthen your neck and pull your head up toward the ceiling. At the same time, press the sitting bones of your buttocks back and away into the seat. Softly engage your abdomen and use your back's strength to stay upright. If needed, use a pillow or rolled-up towel between the back of the seat and your lower spine.

If you still feel uncomfortable after doing this, then try these postures. They will gently massage and soothe your colon:

## CHILD'S POSE

**Refer to page 74 for the details in doing this pose.**

1. Start out in Child's Pose (Photo A), holding it for about a minute.

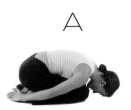

A

## HALF LOCUST
## (ARDHA SALABHASANA)

**Refer to pages 51–52 for the details in doing this pose.**

2. Come on to all fours and then lie down on your belly. Slide your arms under your body. Place your chin on the floor. Lift your right leg (Photo B). Hold for 15 seconds. Repeat on your left leg. Rest.

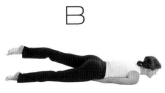

B

### FULL LOCUST (*SALABHASANA*)

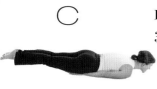

**Refer to pages 53–54 for the details in doing this pose.**

3. With your arms still tucked under your body, lift both legs (Photo C). Hold for about 15–30 seconds.

### FULL FORWARD BEND (*PASCHIMOTANASANA*)

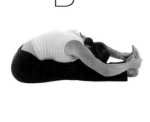

**Refer to pages 68–69 for the details in doing this pose.**

4. Gently turn over onto your back. Bend your knees and roll over to the side. Use your arms to bring yourself up to a seated position. Extend your legs forward and come into a Full Forward Bend (Photo D).

### SUPINE SPINAL TWIST (*JATHARA PARIVARTANASANA*)

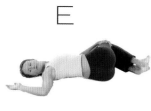

**Refer to pages 94–95 for the details in doing this pose.**

5. Lie down your back. Bend your knees, bring them toward your chest, then let them fall to the left while you look to your right (Photo E). Hold for 45 seconds to 1 minute. Repeat on the opposite side.

### CORPSE POSE (*SAVASANA*)

**Refer to pages 98–99 for the details in doing this pose.**

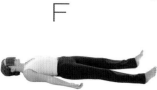

6. Release and lie in a Corpse Pose (Photo F) for a few breaths. You can use an eye pillow while you rest. When you are done, bend your knees and roll over onto your side. Come into any comfortable seated position. Rest easily for a few minutes.

# SIGHTSEEING FATIGUE

You can log in a lot of mileage while walking and exploring a new place. The areas you need to attend to are your lower back, legs, ankles, and feet.

## "MOUNTAIN" WALKING

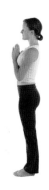

Posture is just as important, if not more so, when you're walking as when you are sitting. It can prevent backaches and knee strain.

Be sure to walk as if you're holding a Mountain Pose (*Tadasana*): ankles, knees, hips, and shoulders in line, chin parallel to the ground, spine long. Take easy strides with open, broad feet. Let your arms swing comfortably.

### Stretch Break

On long treks, stop every 1–2 miles to do this mini-routine:

## CRESCENT MOON

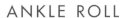

**Refer to pages 138–139 for the details in doing this pose.**

1. Inhale as you elongate your spine (Photo A). Exhale as you stretch to the right (Photo B). Come back to center. Inhale, elongate. Exhale, stretch to the left (Photo C). Do this a few times.

## ANKLE ROLL

2. Using a wall or fence for support, slowly rotate your right ankle in both directions. Then do the same with your left ankle.

## HIP AND CALF LOOSENER

3. Still using the wall or fence, swing your right leg from front to back as if there were a hinge at your hip. Now imagine that hinge at your right knee and let your right calf swing front to back. Repeat for your left hip and calf.

## MODIFIED DOWNWARD FACING DOG

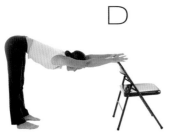

D

4. Find a table, bench, chair, or fence that's about as high as your waist. Stand in front of the support with your legs about hip-width apart. Laying your palms down, hinge forward from your hips, aligning your hips over your feet (Photo D). Keep your back flat and breathe into the stretch in the backs of your legs. This stretch is good for lower backache and discomfort in the shins and calves.

## EAGLE POSTURE (*GARUDASANA*)

E

**Refer to pages 88–89 for the details in doing this pose.**

5. Stand comfortably. Raise your arms above your head. As you lower them, swing your right arm underneath your left arm, intertwining your forearms and bringing your palms together with thumbs toward your face (Photo E). Lift your elbows up to shoulder height.

6. Bend your knees deeply as if you were sitting on a chair. Hoist your right leg over your left. If you can, wrap your right foot back around your left

calf. Repeat steps 5 and 6 with your left arm underneath your right arm and your left leg over your right leg. This stretch is especially good for shinsplints.

## STIFF NECK

If you have a stiff neck after being wedged into a tight seat, or from sleeping in an unfamiliar bed, incorporate the following neck stretching routine into your yoga session. Listen to your body—if it hurts to do any of these stretches, then ease up considerably.

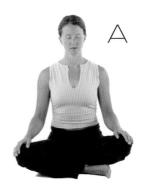

## SIMPLE SITTING POSE (*SUKHASANA*)

**Refer to pages 32–33 for the details in doing this pose.**

1. Sit in Simple Sitting Pose (Photo A), or on a chair with your feet flat on the floor. Allow your spine to lengthen; press your sitting bones down.

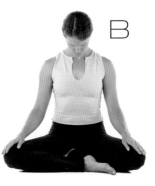

### NECK ROLL

2. Lower the chin toward the chest and hold for three deep breaths (Photo B). Let the head float back up on an inhalation. Repeat a few times.

3. Lift your chin toward the ceiling, stretching your throat (Photo C). Hold for three to five breaths, then lower down.

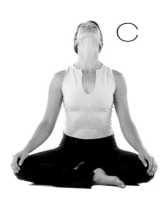

4. Allow your left ear to lower over your left shoulder. Breathe deeply for three to five breaths. Repeat on the right side.

## ACHING BACK

Backaches, like headaches, can have many causes. Chronic back problems need to be diagnosed and treated individually. Yoga can actually make a chronic back problem worse. If you have severe symptoms or a history of back surgery or back problems, consult a physician about what yoga stretches may help and which may hurt.

The occasional backache—caused by improper standing or sitting, or too much walking—can be eased with the following routine.

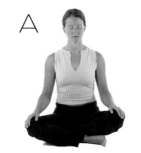

## SIMPLE SITTING POSE (*SUKHASANA*)

**Refer to pages 32–33 for the details in doing this pose.**

1. Sit mindfully for a few minutes (Photo A). If you need support, lean your back against a wall.

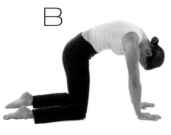

## CAT-COW

**Refer to pages 40–41 for the details in doing this pose.**

2. Slowly make your way to all fours for Cat-Cow. Be careful not to over-arch your back. Keep your spine long. Use the Cat-Cow (Photos B and C) exercise to investigate the sensations in your spine, shoulders, neck, and knees, with special attention to where you may be feeling sensitive in your back area. Continue doing Cat-Cow for about a minute.

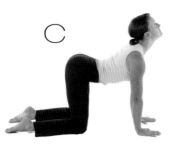

## CHILD'S POSE

**Refer to page 74 for the details in doing this pose.**

3. Come back to a neutral spine and sit back on your heels (Photo D). Round your back and direct your breath to your lower back region. Feel the base of your spine broadening. Stay here for another 30 seconds, breathing steadily.

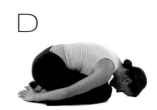

## DOWNWARD FACING DOG

**Refer to page 46 for the details in doing this pose.**

4. Come back up onto all fours. Walk your hands forward about a hand's length, and curl your toes under. Lift your hips up and back as you come into Downward Facing Dog (Photo E). Allow your feet to be hip-width or wider (the wider your legs, the more relief for your back).

5. Explore your Downward Dog. Extend your arms, energize the backs of your legs, breathe into your lower back. Bend your knees and lift your tailbone up even higher to stretch your spine. Be in Downward Dog for as long as it is comfortable for you, and then come back down to Child's Pose to rest and steady your breath.

## THE COBRA (*BHUJANGASANA*)

**Refer to pages 49–50 for the details in doing this pose.**

6. Come back to all fours and slowly walk your hands forward until you are lying on your

abdomen. Let your whole body sink into the
floor with your head turned to one side and
your arms alongside your body, palms up.

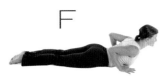

7. Bring your palms to the floor under your
   shoulders for a variation of The Cobra
   (*Bhujangasana;* Photo F). To protect your back,
   separate your legs at least hip-width apart. Be
   sure to keep your buttocks engaged, your legs
   strong, and your kneecaps facing the floor.
   Don't let your legs roll over to the side.

8. Instead of coming up and holding the position,
   inhale and extend your spine forward,
   lifting up head, neck, and chest for the length
   of your inhalation. As you exhale, slowly
   release down and turn your head to the side.
   Continue in this vein for another five breaths,
   turning your head to the opposite side each
   time you lower down.

## MODIFIED FULL LOCUST
## (*SALABHASANA*)

**Refer to pages 53–54 for the details in doing the
unmodified pose.**

9. Remain on your abdomen with your forehead
   on the floor and legs about hip-width apart,
   toes pointed back. Extend your arms overhead
   on the floor, alongside your ears. Gently
   contract your abdomen.

10. Inhale, stretch your right arm forward and your left leg back while keeping your head down and neck long. On the next inhalation, lift your right arm and left leg off the ground, extending your fingertips and toes away from each other. Hold for another breath. On an exhalation, lower down. Repeat with the opposite arm and leg, then repeat the entire cycle again, holding for longer if you are comfortable.

## SUPINE SPINAL TWIST
### (JATHARA PARIVARTANASANA)

**Refer to pages 94–95 for the details in doing this pose.**

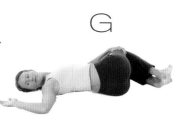

11. Roll onto your back. Bring your hips to one side of your body as you look to the other (Photo G). Hold for 30–60 seconds. Repeat on the other side.

## FULL FORWARD BEND
### (PASCHIMOTANASANA)

**Refer to pages 68–69 for the details in doing this pose.**

12. Come back up on your sitting bones. Bring both feet together and, bending from the waist, fold over (Photo H). Hold for about a minute.

**NOTE:** If a Full Forward Bend is uncomfortable for your back, then spread your legs wide open and come down only a few inches (Photo I).

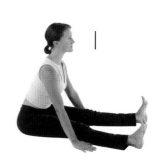

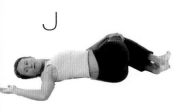

## SUPINE SPINAL TWIST (*JATHARA PARIVARTANASANA*)

**Refer to pages 94–95 for the details in doing this pose.**

13. Lie on your back and hug your knees to your chest. Bring your hips to one side of your body as you look to the other (Photo J). Hold for 30–60 seconds. Repeat on the other side.

## YOGIC SLEEP (*YOGA NIDRA*)

**Refer to pages 100–104 for the details in doing this pose.**

14. Finish up with a session of Yogic Sleep. Allow the deep relaxation to heal your lower back.

## COLDS

A daily yoga practice (and a calm acceptance of life's ups and downs) can fortify your immune system so that you get sick less often. Sometimes traveling can undo that peace of mind and the result is a cold.

The yogic strategy for colds is to hold postures that open your heart. This promotes healing in the bronchial tubes, which prevents further infection in that area. Postures that massage the internal organs are also good because they help squeeze out toxins. But you should avoid forward bends that change the pressure in your head. Most of all, you want your practice to be easygoing and slow to encourage healing.

## EYE MOVEMENTS
## (*NETRA VYAAYAAMAM*)

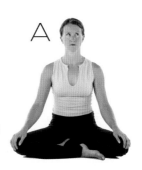

**Refer to page 35 for the details in doing this pose.**

1. Start your practice with some easy Eye Movements to open up your eyes and face (Photos A and B). Spend a little more time than usual massaging your face to relieve sinus-related aches.

## SUN SALUTATION
## (*SURYA NAMASKAR*)

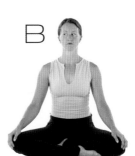

**Refer to pages 42–48 for the details of each position in Sun Salutation.**

2. Move slowly through each of the Sun Salutation positions, beginning with a mindful Mountain Pose (*Tadasana;* Photo C).

3. Position Two: Arms Up (Photo D).

4. Position Three: Forward Bend (*Uttanasana;* Photos E, F, and G).

5. Position Four: Lunge (Photo H).

6. Position Five: Downward Facing Dog (Photo I).

7. Position Six: Knees, Chest, Chin (Photo J).

8. Position Seven: Cobra (Photo K).

9. Position Eight: Downward Facing Dog (Photo L).

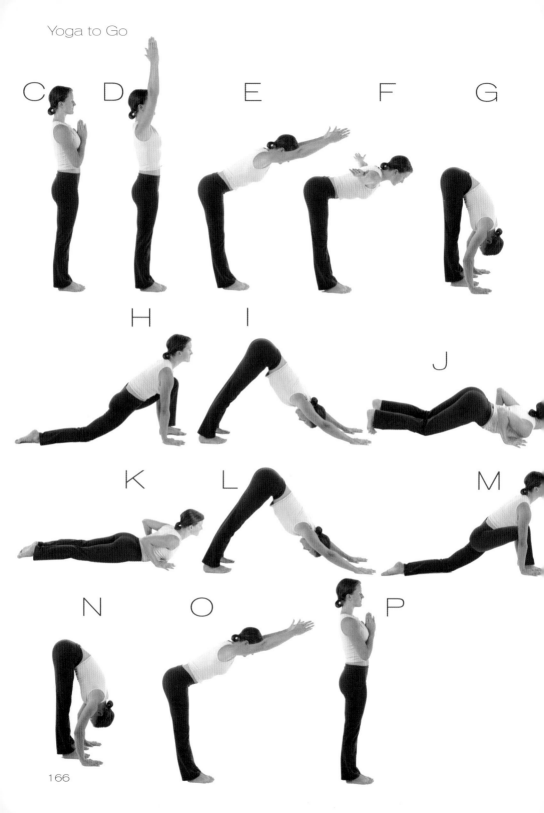

10. Position Nine: Lunge (Photo M).

11. Position Ten: Forward Bend (*Uttanasana;* Photo N).

12. Position Eleven: Reverse Dive (Photo O).

13. Position Twelve: Mountain Pose (*Tadasana;* Photo P). Do one or two more slow and easy rounds.

## CORPSE POSE (*SAVASANA*)

**Refer to pages 98–99 for the details in doing this pose.**

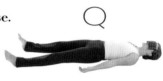

14. Lie down in Corpse Pose (Photo Q) for a few deep breaths. You can use an eye pillow while you rest.

## THE COBRA (*BHUJANGASANA*)

**Refer to pages 49–50 for the details in doing this pose.**

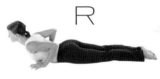

15. Roll onto your abdomen and do two rounds of Cobra Pose (Photo R).

## FULL LOCUST (*SALABHASANA*)

**Refer to pages 53–54 for the details in doing this pose.**

16. Remaining on your abdomen, now do two rounds of Full Locust (Photo S).

## THE BOW (*DHANURASANA*)

**Refer to pages 55–57 for the details in doing this pose.**

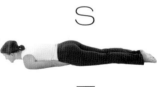

17. Grabbing hold of your ankles, feet, toes, or pant legs, do two rounds of The Bow (Photo T).

## BRIDGE POSE (*SETU BANDHASANA*)

**Refer to pages 61–62 for the details in doing this pose.**

U

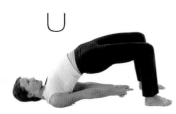

18. Roll over onto your back and hug your knees
to your chest. With your knees bent, lower
the soles of your feet to the floor. Line up your
feet, hips, and knees about hip-width apart.
Then do two rounds of Bridge Pose (Photo U).

## FULL FORWARD BEND (*PASCHIMOTANASANA*)

**Refer to pages 68–69 for the details in doing this pose.**

V

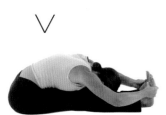

19. If your head is pounding or you are feeling
extremely congested, then go to step 20.
Otherwise, come to sit on your sitting bones,
bring your legs together, and fold over into an
easy Full Forward Bend (Photo V). Hold for
60 seconds.

## LEGS UP THE WALL (*VIPARITA KARANI*)

**Refer to page 81 for the details in doing this pose.**

W

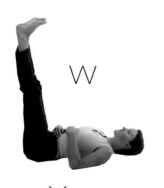

20. Find a free wall and rest your legs up against
the wall (Photo W). Focus on your breath for
about 2 minutes.

## HALF SPINAL TWIST (*ARDHA MATSYENDRASANA*)

**Refer to pages 96–97 for the details in doing this pose.**

X

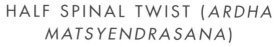

21. Come back into a seated posture with your
legs extended out in front of you. Bring your
right leg over your left and twist to the right

(Photo X). Be sure to keep your stomach relaxed so that the twist can squeeze out the toxins from your digestive tract.

## YOGIC SLEEP (*YOGA NIDRA*)

**Refer to pages 100–104 for the details in doing this pose.**

22. Lie down on your back and take some time for Yogic Sleep.

## RAPID DIAPHRAGMATIC BREATHING (*KAPALABHATI*)

**Refer to page 106 for the details in doing this pose.**

23. Upon "awakening," try practicing up to three rounds of Rapid Diaphragmatic Breathing. Have plenty of tissues handy! Do not force your breath. If you are too congested and your breath isn't coming easily, then just sit and practice the Deep Three-Part Breath (*Dirga Swasam*; see pages 104–105).

24. End your practice by chanting "OM" slowly and pitched deeply to massage the inner core of your body.

## DEPRESSION

Travel can exhilarate and stimulate. For some people, seeing new places is the greatest joy in life. For others, particularly business travelers, it may be a lonely, dull, or disillusioning experience.

Yoga postures can help bring the luster back to your mind and body. Choose postures that open your heart and stimulate your adrenal glands. It is better to do them at a slightly more vigorous pace in order to wake up the stagnant energies in your body. You want to be even more diligent than usual about keeping your mind on the present moment rather than stuck in the past or fantasizing about the

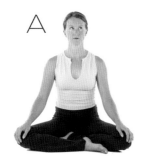

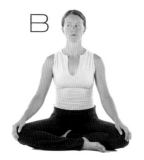

future. You want your practice to be about discovering the joy of the present, not striving for some far-off experience.

During this practice, make a commitment to keeping your eyes open. Try to literally let the light into your brain. Closing your eyes can be soothing, but it may also cause you to dwell on sad thoughts.

## EYE MOVEMENTS
### (*NETRA VYAAYAAMAM*)

**Refer to page 35 for the details in doing this pose.**

1. Mindfully and slowly circle your eyes in a clockwise direction (Photos A and B). Do this several times, then move your eyes in a counterclockwise direction.

## SUN SALUTATION
### (*SURYA NAMASKAR*)

**Refer to pages 42–48 for the details of each position in Sun Salutation.**

2. Move energetically through each of the Sun Salutation positions, beginning with Position One: Mountain Pose (*Tadasana;* Photo C).

3. Position Two: Arms Up (Photo D).

4. Position Three: Forward Bend (*Uttanasana;* Photos E, F, and G).

5. Position Four: Lunge (Photo H).

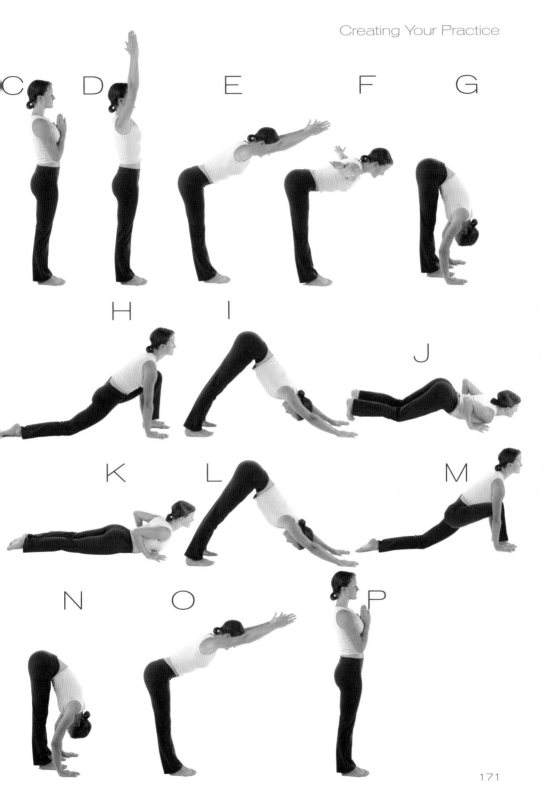

6. Position Five: Downward Facing Dog (Photo I).

7. Position Six: Knees, Chest, Chin (Photo J).

8. Position Seven: Cobra (Photo K).

9. Position Eight: Downward Facing Dog (Photo L). Hold for three full breaths.

10. Position Nine: Lunge (Photo M).

11. Position Ten: Forward Bend (*Uttanasana;* Photo N).

12. Position Eleven: Reverse Dive (Photo O).

13. Position Twelve: Mountain Pose (*Tadasana;* Photo P). Repeat the Sun Salutation four to eight more times.

## WARRIOR I (VIRABHADRASANA I)

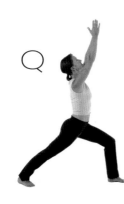

**Refer to pages 82–84 for the details in doing this pose.**

14. Take a wide stance and hold Warrior I (Photo Q) for 30–45 seconds on each side. Keep your chest open and lifted through to Warrior II and Triangle Pose. Feel the power and rootedness of your legs.

# WARRIOR II (*VIRABHADRASANA II*)

**Refer to pages 84–85 for the details in doing this pose.**

15. Open into Warrior II (Photo R) and hold for 30–45 seconds on each side. Find your breath and focus on it as your spine lengthens.

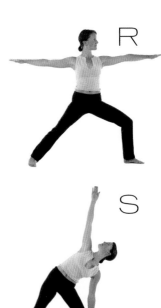

# TRIANGLE (*TRIKONASANA*)

**Refer to pages 86–87 for the details in doing this pose.**

16. Straighten your front leg and slide into Triangle Pose (Photo S). Hold for 30–45 seconds on each side.

# THE COBRA (*BHUJANGASANA*)

**Refer to pages 49–50 for the details in doing this pose.**

17. Now lie down on your abdomen. Position your hands on the floor underneath your shoulders and lift yourself into the Cobra (Photo T). Concentrate on your heart lifting and collarbones separating. Keep your eyes lifted up toward the ceiling. Hold for 15 seconds. Release, then repeat.

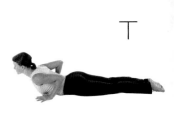

# THE BOW (*DHANURASANA*)

**Refer to pages 55–57 for the details in doing this pose.**

18. Still lying on your abdomen, grab whatever part of your leg you feel comfortable holding and lift both parts of your body (Photo U). Again, concentrate on your heart lifting and hold for 15 seconds. Release, then repeat.

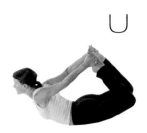

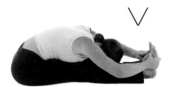

## FULL FORWARD BEND (*PASCHIMOTANASANA*)

**Refer to pages 68–69 for the details in doing this pose.**

19. Remain on the floor, but come to sit on your sitting bones. Bring your legs together and fold over into a Full Forward Bend (Photo V). Hold for 30–60 seconds. See if you can keep your eyes open the whole time.

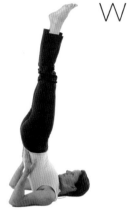

## SHOULDER STAND (*SARVANGASANA*)

**Refer to pages 76–78 for the details in doing this pose.**

20. Lie back down and come into a Shoulder Stand (Photo W). Try holding your pose for at least 2 minutes.

## THE FISH (*MATSYASANA*)

**Refer to pages 58–60 for the details in doing this pose.**

21. With your legs together, move your pelvis toward your feet and lift your rib cage high up into the air. Arch your upper body. Let your head relax back and lower the top of your head to the floor (Photo X). Hold for as long as you feel comfortable. Release and lie in Corpse Pose.

## SUPINE SPINAL TWIST (*JATHARA PARIVARTANASANA*)

**Refer to pages 94–95 for the details in doing this pose.**

22. After you come out of Fish Pose, lie down on the floor for a second, then take a

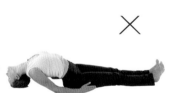

leisurely Supine Spinal Twist (Photo Y). Hold for at least 30–60 seconds. Repeat on the other side.

## YOGIC SLEEP AND CORPSE POSE

**Refer to pages 100–104 for Yogic Sleep and pages 98–99 for Corpse Pose.**

23. Lie back down on your back and come in Yogic Sleep (Photo Z). If you don't have the time for Yogic Sleep, then lie in Corpse Pose for at least 5 minutes. You can use an eye pillow while you rest.

## RAPID DIAPHRAGMATIC BREATHING (*KAPALABHATI*) AND ALTERNATE NOSTRIL BREATHING (*NADI SUDHI*)

**Refer to page 106 for Rapid Diaphragmatic Breathing and pages 106–107 for Alternate Nostril Breathing.**

24. Upon awakening, take three rounds of Rapid Diaphragmatic Breathing for energy and then about 3 minutes of Alternate Nostril Breathing to balance the hemispheres of your brain.

### *Yogic Insights for Depression*

It may help to explore the thoughts and beliefs behind your feelings through journaling. A yogic approach to depression balances *asana* and breathing (*pranayama*) practice with insight. You might start by contemplating the qualities of *santosa* and *tapas* (see pages 22–23). Low moods sometimes come from comparing your life with someone else's, or to some fantasy ideal. *Santosa* reminds you that who you are and what you have are enough. *Tapas* reminds you that a calm acceptance of life's low points can help see you through the hard times.

In the *Yoga Sutras*, Patanjali reports, "*yoga citta vritti nirodah*": "yoga is the control of the fluctuations of the mind." Through awareness and practice, you learn that you are not your thoughts—whether they are happy or sad thoughts. You are actually bigger than your thoughts. So the next time you feel down, you might ask yourself: "Who is depressed?" The Universal Self, your true nature, doesn't know how to feel depressed, so it can't be your true nature that's down. The "I" who is feeling depressed is your ego, the part of you that is created to deal with the everyday world. That "I" is a construction of your thoughts—a personality created by choice that can be rearranged by choice, too.

It is important to remember that everybody goes through sad periods and bad days. You don't need to be happy every minute. Good and bad thoughts will pass by you. Give yourself comfort with the perspective that your emotions and thoughts don't define you.

## A FULL 90-MINUTE ROUTINE

If you have the time, here is a complete hatha yoga session. It includes all the basic poses, some chanting, meditation, deep relaxation, and breathing exercises.

### SIMPLE SITTING POSE (*SUKHASANA*) AND DEEP THREE-PART BREATH (*DIRGA SWASAM PRANAYAMA*)

**Refer to pages 32–33 for the details in Simple Sitting Pose and pages 104–105 for Deep Three-Part Breathing.**

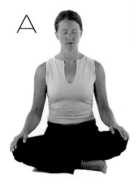

A

1. Start in Simple Sitting Pose (Photo A) and watch your breath. Slowly engage in Deep Three-Part Breathing. Do this for 1–3 minutes, then chant "OM" three times. Allow the sound to vibrate through your solar plexus and head cavity. With your eyes still closed, notice how you feel. Relax your forehead, inhale deeply, and let out a big loud sigh.

## EYE MOVEMENTS (*NETRA VYAAYAAMAM*)

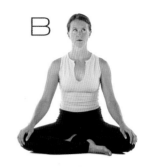

**Refer to page 35 for the details in doing this pose.**

2. Open your eyes and then do a few rounds of Eye Movements (Photos B and C), first in one direction and then the other.

## SHOULDER ROLLS

**Refer to page 38 for the details in doing this pose.**

3. Still sitting comfortably with your legs crossed, do several shoulder rolls.

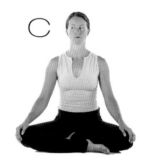

## CAT-COW

**Refer to pages 40–41 for the details in doing this pose.**

4. Come onto your hands and knees. Do Cat-Cow (Photos D and E) for about a minute.

# SUN SALUTATION (*SURYA NAMASKAR*)

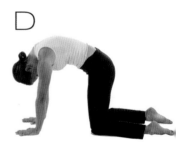

**Refer to pages 42–48 for the details of each position in Sun Salutation.**

5. Perform Position One: Mountain Pose (*Tadasana;* Photo F).

6. Position Two: Arms Up (Photo G).

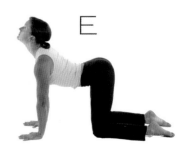

7. Position Three: Forward Bend (*Uttanasana;* Photos H, I, and J).

8. Position Four: Lunge (Photo K).

9. Position Five: Downward Facing Dog (Photo L).

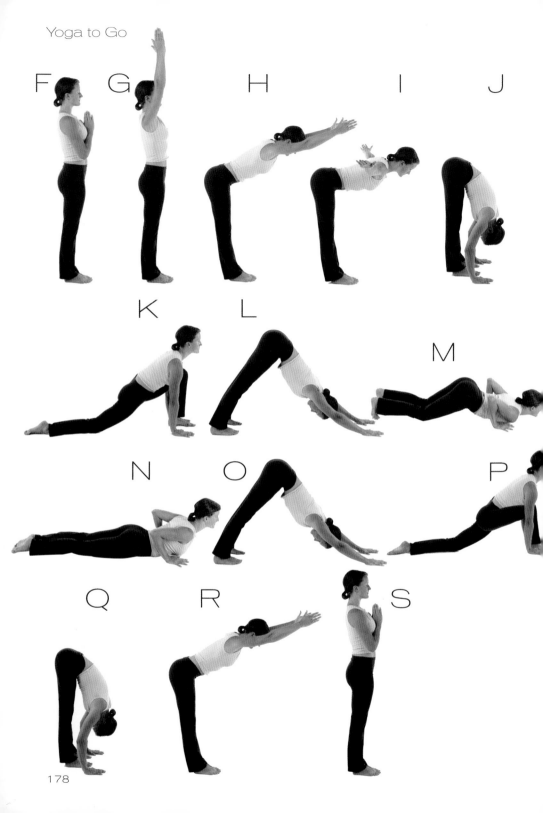

F   G   H   I   J

K   L   M

N   O   P

Q   R   S

10. Position Six: Knees, Chest, Chin (Photo M).

11. Position Seven: Cobra (Photo N).

12. Position Eight: Downward Facing Dog (Photo O).

13. Position Nine: Lunge (Photo P).

14. Position Ten: Forward Bend (Photo Q).

15. Position Eleven: Reverse Dive (Photo R).

16. Position Twelve: Mountain Pose (*Tadasana;* Photo S).

17. Do two more rounds of Sun Salutation.

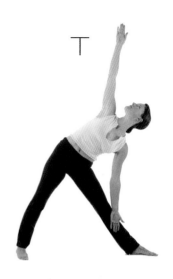

## TRIANGLE (*TRIKONASANA*)

**Refer to pages 86–87 for the details in doing this pose.**

18. Bring your left leg forward, right leg back. Slide into Triangle Pose (Photo T). Hold for 30 seconds. Repeat on the other side.

## TREE (*VRKSASANA*)

**Refer to pages 90–91 for the details in doing this pose.**

19. Come back to stand in Mountain Pose (*Tadasana*). Shift the weight of your body over to your right foot. Bring your left foot to your ankle, calf, or thigh (Photo U). Repeat on the other side.

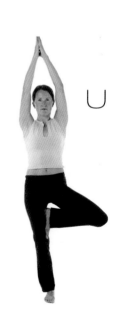

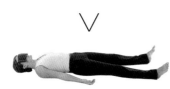

## CORPSE POSE (SAVASANA)

**Refer to pages 98–99 for the details in doing this pose.**

20. Lie down on the floor and rest in Corpse Pose (Photo V) for a minute. You can use an eye pillow while you rest.

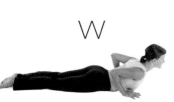

## THE COBRA (BHUJANGASANA)

**Refer to pages 49–50 for the details in doing this pose.**

21. Roll over onto your abdomen. Place your hands underneath your shoulders and come into Cobra Pose (Photo W). Hold for several breaths and then release. Repeat once more.

## HALF LOCUST (ARDHA SALABHASANA)

**Refer to pages 51–52 for the details in doing this pose.**

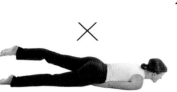

22. Now tuck your arms underneath your body with your palms facing up against your thighs. Lift your right leg up. Hold for several breaths and then release. Repeat on your left leg (Photo X), then repeat once more for each leg.

## FULL LOCUST (SALABHASANA)

**Refer to pages 53–54 for the details in doing this pose.**

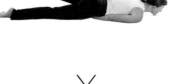

23. With your arms still tucked under you, bring both legs up together (Photo Y). Hold for several breaths and then release. Repeat once more.

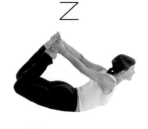

## THE BOW (DHANURASANA)

**Refer to pages 55–57 for the details in doing this pose.**

24. Bend your knees, bring your heels in toward your hips, and reach your hands back to grab

hold of your legs wherever you can comfortably reach: the ankles, feet, toes, or pant legs. As you inhale, lift the front and back parts of your body (Photo Z). Hold for several breaths and then release. Repeat once more.

## CHILD'S POSE (*BALASANA*)

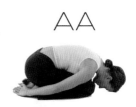

**Refer to pages 74–75 for the details in doing this pose.**

25. Place your hands on the floor under your shoulders and push back into Child's Pose (Photo AA). Breathe into your lower back.

## DIAMOND POSE (*VAJRASANA*)

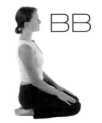

**Refer to page 34 for the details in doing this pose.**

26. Slowly roll up one vertebra at a time and then sit back on your heels (Photo BB).

## THE STAFF POSE (*DANDASANA*)

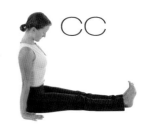

**Refer to pages 63–64 for the details in doing this pose.**

27. Let your hips spill over to the side and draw your legs out in front of you (Photo CC). Pull your buttock flesh out, bring your legs together, and flex your feet flexed.

## HEAD-TO-KNEE POSE (*JANUSIRSHASANA*)

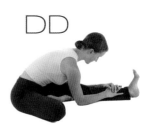

**Refer to pages 65–67 for the details in doing this pose.**

28. Bend your right knee and open it to the side with the sole of your right foot against the inside of your left leg. Fold over (Photo DD). Hold for several breaths and then release. Repeat on your left leg.

## FULL FORWARD BEND (*PASCHIMOTANASANA*)

**EE**

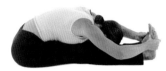

**Refer to pages 68–69 for the details in doing this pose.**

29. Now draw both legs out together in front of you. Folding from your waist, extend your upper body out and over your legs (Photo EE). Hold for several breaths.

## SHOULDER STAND (*SARVANGASANA*)

**FF**

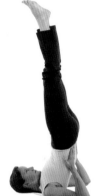

**Refer to pages 76–78 for the details in doing this pose.**

30. Lie on your back and bring your knees into your chest. Release your back to the floor. Softly rock from side to side, massaging your spine.

31. When you are ready, bring your legs over your head and then come into a Shoulder Stand (Photo FF). Hold for 45 seconds to 1 minute.

## THE FISH (*MATSYASANA*)

**Refer to pages 58–60 for the details in doing this pose.**

32. Come down from Shoulder Stand and lie on the floor for a second. When you are ready, bring the crown of your head to the floor and lift your rib cage high up into the air (Photo GG). Hold for 30–45 seconds.

**GG**

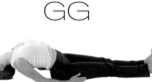

## CORPSE POSE (*SAVASANA*)

**Refer to pages 98–99 for the details in doing this pose.**

33. Release from Fish Pose. Roll your head from side to side and bring your knees into your chest to release any back tension. Then lie in

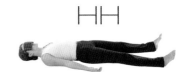

Corpse Pose (Photo HH) for a moment. You can use an eye pillow while you rest.

## HALF SPINAL TWIST (*ARDHA MATSYENDRASANA*)

**Refer to pages 96–97 for the details in doing this pose.**

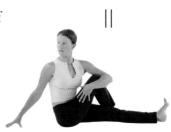

34. Bend your knees and take hold of the backs of your thighs. Rock yourself into a seated position. Extend your legs out in front of you. Bend your right leg and bring it over your left leg. Twist to the right (Photo II). Hold for several breaths and then switch sides.

## YOGA MUDRA

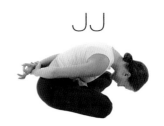

**Refer to pages 111–112 for the details in doing this pose.**

35. Come back into a simple cross-legged position for Yoga Mudra (Photo JJ).

## CORPSE POSE AND YOGIC SLEEP

**Refer to pages 98–104 for the details in doing these poses.**

36. Lie in Corpse Pose (Photo KK) for a few minutes and then transition into Yogic Sleep. Either follow your recording of the instructions or just use your intuition and memory to guide you through the stages of release. Using an eye pillow can help you settle deeper into the stages. Pay special attention to tightening and then releasing the areas where you feel tension. Remember not to fall asleep.

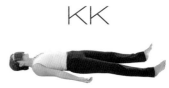

## DEEP THREE-PART BREATH (*DIRGA SWASAM PRANAYAMA*), RAPID DIAPHRAGMATIC BREATHING (*KAPALABHATI*), AND ALTERNATE NOSTRIL BREATHING (*NADI SUDHI PRANAYAMA*)

**Refer to pages 104–105 for the detailed steps in Deep Three-Part Breath, page 106 for Rapid Diaphragmatic Breathing, and pages 106–107 for Alternate Nostril Breathing.**

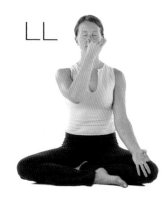

LL

37. Take your time coming back into a seated position. Slowly lift your body up one vertebra at a time, bringing your head up last. Reserve about 5 minutes for breathing exercises in this order: Deep Three-Part Breath (*Dirga Swasam Pranayama*) followed by Rapid Diaphragmatic Breathing (*Kapalabhati*), then Alternate Nostril Breathing (*Nadi Sudhi Pranayama;* Photo LL).

## MEDITATION AND CONTEMPLATION

**Refer to Chapter Five for more details.**

38. Sit quietly and peacefully, and observe your breath. If any thoughts or feelings arise, let them pass by you like the clouds in the sky. Sit for as long as you can, then close your practice with three more rounds of "OM."

When I travel, a lifesaver for me is to use two tennis balls tied into a sock. I use this as a self-massage tool up and down my back to release compression after a long plane travel. It's cheap, very effective, and small enough to fit into my luggage.

What I also find extremely relaxing is to weave seed beads. This takes up all my concentration so that the hours pass by to my great pleasure. If I do not need to do work on a plane, I will think of a good friend or acquaintance, a student or host who has been very supportive to me, or someone who is ill or having a difficult time in their life as I design a bracelet or necklace for them. I think about how nice it would feel for them to receive something special. As I am beading, I dwell on lovingkindness towards this person. To me, this is as good as a formal lovingkindness meditation.

—Donna Farhi, registered movement therapist, yoga teacher, and author of *The Breathing Book: Good Health and Vitality Through Essential Breath Work* and *Yoga Mind, Body & Spirit: A Return to Wholeness* (Henry Holt & Company, Inc.)

### Creating Your Own Practice

If none of the routines or stretches described in this chapter speaks to you, use what you've learned about the postures and their individual benefits in Chapter 2 to design a sequence that meets your needs. Let your intuition guide you. Aim for balance: even if you're emphasizing, for example, back bends to energize your body, your body will need a few forward bends tossed in. Remember that Sun Salutation (see pages 42–48) is a complete routine that stretches all the major muscle groups.

More important than learning the postures or memorizing routines is to simply keep in mind that your True Nature is peace and pure consciousness. Remember that, and your journey should be a joyous one.

# CHAPTER FOUR

# Eating Well on the Road

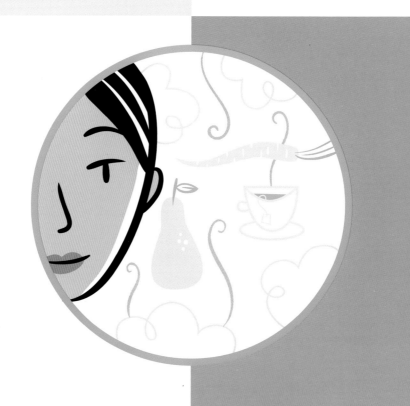

Yoga is not for the person who eats too much,

nor for the one who fasts excessively.

—*The Bhagavad Gita*

Healthy eating is just as important as any other part of your yoga practice. A good diet promotes peace of mind, strength, and ease of body. What you take into your body, and your attitude towards eating, influences the content and flavor of your thoughts. Ancient yogic texts, such as the *Hatha Yoga Pradipika*, provide dietary guidelines and insights into foods and their energy (or *gunas*).

## THE GUNAS

The yoga tradition identifies three main types of energy (or *gunas*) at play in the universe: *sattwa* (purity), *tamas* (inertia, heaviness), and *rajas* (action). These energies manifest everywhere and in everything, to varying degrees, including the food you eat.

*Tamasic* food is heavy, oily, overcooked food—or an excess of food in general—that promotes sluggishness. *Rajasic* food is spicy food

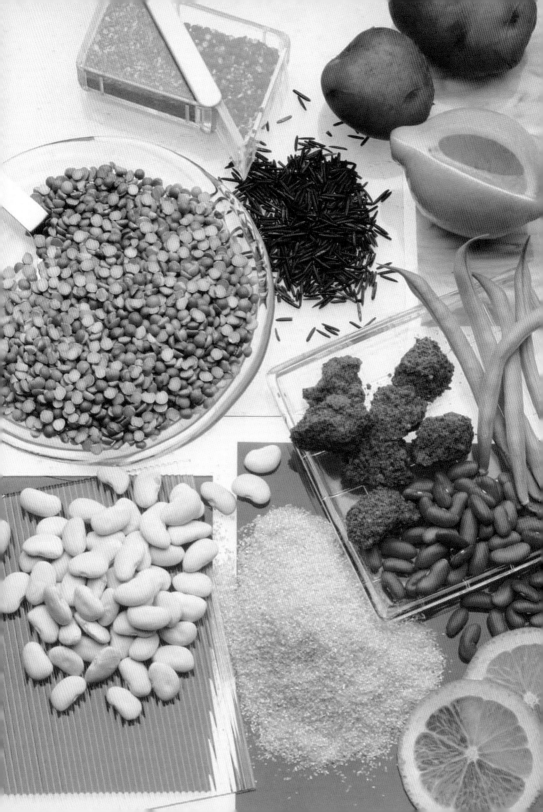

that excites your senses and revs up your mind, or it can be food that is eaten too fast or while you are on the go. *Sattwic* food is light, fresh, nourishing, and easily digestible food that is consumed in moderate amounts and at restful moments.

*Sattwic* foods include most fruits, nuts, vegetables, and whole grains as well as honey, pure water, and milk. A *sattwic* diet is a purifying diet that promotes clear thinking and a calm, even frame of mind—just what a traveler needs to maintain balance. *Sattwic* eating means taking nourishment in order to be strong and purposeful rather than solely for sensual gratification or as a distraction from boredom or anxiety. This doesn't mean that food isn't to be enjoyed. Eating can be one of the simplest and most satisfying pleasures of life. But the enjoyment arises from feeling nourished rather than from the gross effects of the flavor of the food.

*Sattwic* eating is done slowly and consciously, without rushing. You neither overeat nor starve yourself. You breathe consciously as you eat and pay attention to your meal rather than eat while you are doing something else, such as watching TV or reading the newspaper. As a *sattwic* eater, you gratefully honor the lifeforce in the food and the gift it gives you.

*Sattwic* eating also means having your meals at regular times. A consistent eating routine during the whirlwind of traveling can have a positive effect on your digestion and overall well-being. Try to eat your biggest meal at lunch, when your digestive fire is strongest. A heavy dinner can give you an uncomfortable night's sleep.

## THE SATTWIC DIET

A *sattwic* diet is understood to be vegetarian. Don't panic. This does not mean that, in order to practice yoga, you have to suddenly cut meat and eggs from your diet. But it may be a strategy to consider, even temporarily.

A basic vegetarian, low-fat regimen is supported by the USDA, the World Health Organization, and the American Dietetic Association. It is also the best diet to support overtaxed traveling bodies. Making even an interim commitment to eating vegetarian is a positive step. It can keep you from sleepwalking into whatever fast-food restaurant happens to be available. As meat is a staple of the fast-food industry, avoiding their fat-laden and over-processed foods, which are associated with the *tamas* and *rajas* energies, can produce many benefits for your body and mind.

However, if eating vegetarian seems like too big or stressful a step to take, simply consider cutting out processed foods from your diet. Choose lean meat and fish as your protein source. But above all, use your intuition. The more you practice yoga, the more sensitive you become to your body's deep needs. If eating a vegetarian diet feels right to you, follow through on that and learn to eat a vegetarian diet that will nourish you as much as a nonvegetarian diet. If the choice to eat vegetarian doesn't feel right for you, then listen to that guidance.

Following a *sattwic* diet, or semi-*sattwic* diet, on the road is becoming increasingly easier to do these days. As the general public becomes more health conscious, healthful dining can be found in unexpected places like airports, train stations, and roadside diners. In the late 1990s, the American Dietetic Association investigated two dozen random airports across the United States and found that 40% of them featured salad bars while 92% had fresh salads available. Fresh fruit, fresh fruit juices, and low-fat yogurt were also readily available at all the airports studied.

When ordering from a menu, try to keep *sattwic*: fresh, light, whole-grains rather than white or processed flours. Try to select foods that are fat-free—and remember to eat slowly and sparingly.

If you're planning on bringing your own food for "quality assurance" purposes, vegetarian food packs and keeps well on the road.

## A LIST OF *SATTWIC* FOODS

**DAIRY:** Butter, Buttermilk, Homemade Cheese, Milk, Yogurt

**GRAINS:** Barley, Rice, Millet, Quinoa, Buckwheat, Cornmeal, Soybeans, Oats, Whole Wheat

**NUTS/LEGUMES:** Almonds, Sunflower Seeds, Cashews, Lentils, Bean Sprouts, Brazil Nuts, Peas, Macadamia Nuts, Mung Beans

**VEGETABLES:** Beets, Carrots, Cucumbers, All Green Leafy Vegetables, Sweet Potatoes, Squash, Turnips

**FRUITS:** Apples, Bananas, Coconuts, Dates, Grapes, Melons, Mangos, Oranges, Plums, Pomegranates

## WHEN IN DOUBT, GO "ETHNIC"

The safest bet for a light vegetable-rich meal is to eat Chinese, Italian, Middle Eastern, or Indian food. Most Chinese take-out places offer a "health" or "diet" menu—or you can request a meal of steamed veggies and tofu (or chicken). Order brown rice if it's on the menu, or at least skip the fried rice and take a small serving of white.

Italian restaurants, of course, will have a variety of pasta dishes to choose from. Pasta primavera with a simple marinara or garlic-and-oil sauce and a tossed green salad on the side should be easy to get in even the most casual Italian eatery. Ask if the minestrone has a meat-broth base. If not, you've got a nutritious one-bowl meal.

Middle Eastern dining features healthy vegetarian options like tabbouleh (bulgur wheat, onions, tomatoes and lots of parsley), hummus (chickpeas and tahini), baba ghanoush (eggplant dip), and falafel (chickpea balls with cilantro, garlic and cumin).

Indian fare leans towards vegetarian, although the food is often cooked in ghee (clarified butter) and can be on the oily side. Ask if you can have your meal steamed, braised, or cooked in water.

## SATTWA IN THE SKY

High altitudes and pressurized airplane cabins deplete your body of water and oxygen. In addition to keeping *sattwic*, you need to address that depletion by staying hydrated and oxygenated.

When flying, bottled water or fruit juice (especially orange, which bolsters oxygen-transporting red blood cells) are much better choices than soft drinks or alcohol. Soda often contains high amounts of sodium and caffeine, which dry out the body. Alcohol also dehydrates the body and clouds the mind.

Zinc, calcium, iron, B vitamins, and vitamin E can boost oxygen metabolism. Nuts, beans, peas, carrots, and dark green leafy vegetables, like spinach, are rich sources of these vitamins and minerals. Eat them before, during, and after flying.

In-flight meals have become scarcer on commercial airlines since late 2001. This is good news, since in-flight meals are frozen and then reheated, which means that they do not fulfill the first requirement of *sattwa*: freshness. In addition, they can often be fatty, salty, and overprocessed.

If your flight is less than 2 or 3 hours, avoid eating on the plane. While in the air, you won't be moving much, so you will not need much fuel. On shorter flights, food is often just a distraction anyway. When you eat solely for recreational purposes, you're disregarding the *sattwic* principle of "eating to live, not living to eat."

On flights 3 hours or longer, it is best to bring your own food onboard. Fresh fruits and vegetables make good between-meal snacks. Apples, oranges, raw carrots, and raw broccoli pack and keep well while softer fruits and vegetables (such as strawberries, grapes, avocados, pears) are best left at home. Unsalted nuts, trail mix, and low-fat yogurt also make good snacks. It is important to note that if broccoli and fruit give you gas, avoid eating these on airplanes, as the pressurized cabin exacerbates the effects of gas in your intestines.

For easily packable and neat meals, bring sandwiches, whole-grain breakfast cereal (ask your flight attendant for skim milk), whole-grain pasta salad with vegetables, bean salad, or tabbouleh.

If you have a very long flight and cannot bring food with you, then you can call the airline ahead of time to arrange for a "special meal." Most major airlines offer a vegetarian menu, meals for diabetics, "Hindu" dishes, fat-free/low calorie dinners, etc. You can request any of these meals while making your reservations. It's important to confirm this request 2 days prior to your flight and again at the airport check-in. That extra confirmation allows time for any last-minute airport food purchases.

## CHEW-CHEW: EATING ON TRAINS

The quality of food available from dining and buffet cars on trains differs from railway company to railway company, and country to country. But, in general, the same rules for airline food apply to train food. If you want to request a special diet, call a few days ahead. While the quality of food on trains tends to be higher than airplane food, it's still a good idea to bring your own food when you can to ensure freshness. If you happen to be traveling in Europe, your rail station may even have a grocery store on premises where you can buy fresh food and portable meals.

## NUTRITION FOR COMMON TRAVEL AILMENTS
### JET LAG

Studies by the U.S. Department of Energy's Argonne National Laboratory suggest that following a feast/fast diet a few days before your flight may help you overcome the effects of jet lag. The diet states: Three days before your trip, you "feast" by eating a large protein-rich breakfast and lunch and a high-carbohydrate dinner (grains and fruits). The next day, you "fast" on about 700–1000 calories of light and liquidy foods or salads. The

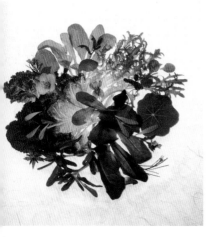

next day, the day before your trip, you "feast" again. On the day of your flight, you eat very lightly and drink lots of water. Upon arriving at your destination, you sync up your meals according to your new time zone.

In addition to drinking plenty of water and staying oxygenated, keep in mind the rule of thumb that protein helps to keep you awake while carbohydrates help you to sleep. If your strategy for avoiding jet lag includes sleeping on international flights, then eat accordingly.

### MOTION SICKNESS

Nausea, cold sweats, and dizziness can occur when using any mode of transportation (see "Nausea or Motion Sickness," pages 149–150). Clinical studies indicate that ginger, in powdered form, may ease the effects of travel nausea. The recommended dose is 500 mg taken about 45 minutes before travel, and then 500 mg every 2 hours if the nausea persists.

Less formal observation shows that ginger in any form can help to settle a queasy stomach. If you experience air sickness, ask your

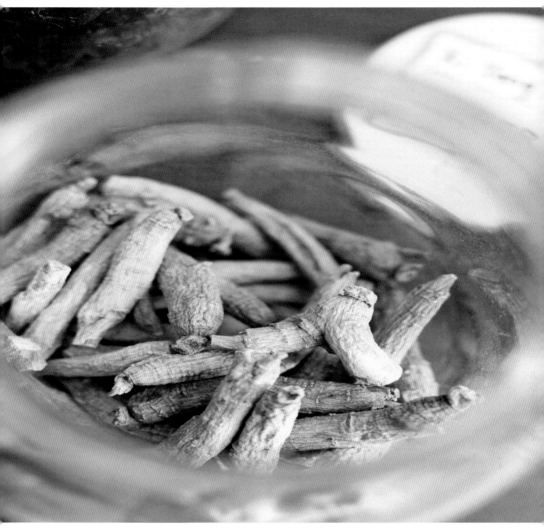

steward for a ginger ale (unless the carbonation makes you feel bloated). You can also bring your own powdered ginger capsules, ginger candy, or pickled ginger.

Nausea also responds well to cool water. You can drink it or simply place it against your forehead as a cold compress. Some people find relief by munching salted crackers and others find that the peppermint taste of chewing gum or breath mints can help calm the stomach.

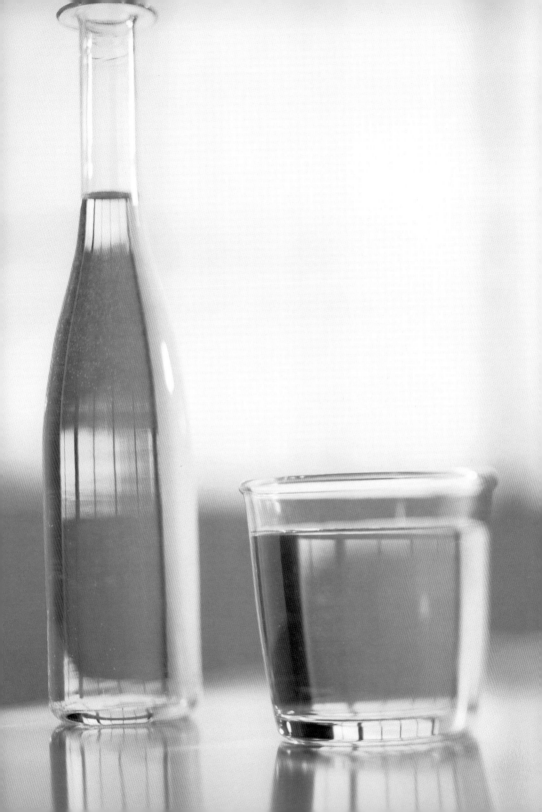

## DIARRHEA

If you are traveling to an area where you may encounter contaminated water and food, you should consult your physician about immunization and antimicrobial drugs. In addition, you should stick to bottled beverages and water boiled and decontaminated with iodine. Finally, avoid eating food sold on the street or in unclean restaurants.

But even with all these precautions, you may still get diarrhea from the food or stress. If you are experiencing severe diarrhea, you may need to find a physician. If your symptoms are less severe, these natural remedies may just do the trick.

When bothered by diarrhea, your body needs light, bland foods, and it needs to regain lost minerals and fluids. Brown rice, bananas, and clear broths (especially miso soup) can help. The pectin found in apples—either eaten whole, or as applesauce or room-temperature juice—is said to have a healing effect on both diarrhea and constipation. Stick to a simple, bland diet until the diarrhea lessens and then slowly start adding more fiber to your diet in the form of whole grains. Drink bottled water or suck on ice chips to help replace lost fluids. Avoid dairy products until you are completely over your diarrhea.

## CONSTIPATION

Travel can create a temporary sedentariness that slows down bowel function. If light exercise or the *asana* routine in Chapter Three (see "Constipation," pages 155–156) doesn't stimulate your sluggish intestines, then try a nutritional approach to the problem.

First, make sure you are getting enough water. Drink at least 64 ounces of water each day. Eat foods rich in both soluble and insoluble fiber. Insoluble fiber includes apples, wheat germ, and wheat bran. Soluble fiber is found in abundance in oat bran and in smaller but good amounts in most vegetables, legumes, and fruits.

The time-honored cure for constipation is prunes, which help stimulate the intestines. If you are prone to constipation when you travel, dried prunes are easy to pack.

## INSOMNIA

The stresses of travel and jet lag can trigger temporary insomnia. Some simple yoga postures (see "A Good Night's Sleep," pages 124–130) and a warm cup of herbal tea can go far in helping you get to sleep. But a peaceful *sattwic* diet will also contribute to a restful sleep.

The first step is eliminating, or at least decreasing, the amount of caffeine and alcohol from your travel diet. Then aim to eat a healthy carbohydrate-rich diet—vegetables, legumes, and whole grains—which helps boost the serotonin levels in your brain that support healthy sleep patterns and relaxation. The production of serotonin is also boosted by an amino acid called L-tryptophan, the ingredient in turkey that induces the blissful feeling of fullness and sleepiness after a big Thanksgiving dinner. Tryptophan can be found in dairy products, bananas, and sunflower seeds.

Another brain chemical that causes sleepiness is melatonin, a hormone produced by the pineal gland. Studies of melatonin taken orally to aid insomnia and jet lag are inconclusive and the side effects are still being studied. However, eating foods that contain naturally occurring, low doses of melatonin is a venerable home remedy. Melatonin can be found in oats, corn, ginger, barley, and bananas.

## ANXIETY

Some of the symptoms of anxiety include jitters, racing heartbeat, negative thinking, and an inability to focus or relax. Hatha yoga greatly reduces anxiety and a *sattwic* diet supports your nervous system to decrease the likelihood of panic attacks and stress. But if you find that you need something extra to cope with temporary travel-induced anxiety, make sure that you are getting enough B and C vitamins in your diet.

Vitamin B6 is an important nutrient. One of its many functions is to help the nervous system run efficiently. You can get healthy doses of B6 in bananas, figs, avocados, potatoes, beans, chickpeas, and oatmeal.

Vitamin B12 aids in the production of healthy nerve cells. Since significant amounts of it are found only in animal products, like poultry and fish, a vegetarian diet may be lacking in vitamin B12. If you've adopted a yogic diet, be sure to consume your vitamin B12 in alternative ways: in dairy products, yogurt, fortified cereals, or vitamin supplements.

Vitamin C, known for its effectiveness in boosting immunity, is a powerful antioxidant. Studies imply that large doses of the vitamin can decrease the level of stress hormones in the blood. Citrus fruits and dark green leafy vegetables provide healthy levels of Vitamin C.

And, finally, never underestimate the calming effects of a nice cup of chamomile tea.

# CHAPTER FIVE

# Travel and Meditation

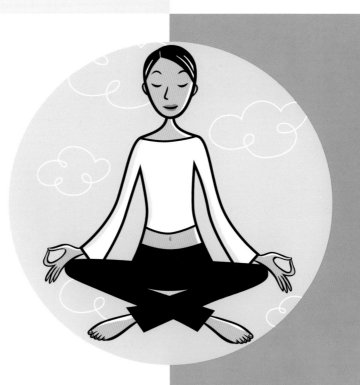

God is with you wherever you go.

—Joshua 1:9


Wherever you go, there you are.

— Peter Weller, *The Adventures of Buckaroo Banzai*


Meditation, or *dhyana*, is the union with your higher self. It's characterized by a transcendence of thought, an utter stillness of the mind, and a peaceful feeling in the body. This happens when you quiet down your rational mind and awaken the resting knowledge of yourself as limitless consciousness. Think of meditation as that inspired moment during a concert when a soloist is on fire and playing music that seems directly channeled from some higher source. Unfortunately, you can't learn that from a book—that inspiration is an unplanned moment of grace. Yet a good performer is more likely to experience those moments by preparing for them with disciplined practice, study, and repetition. In the same way, you can learn some practices that lead up to a meditative state, and provide deep rest for the nervous system on the way there, by doing the daily yogic work of following the *yamas* and *niyamas*, and engaging in the *asanas* (postures), *pranayama* (breathing exercises), and *dhurana* (concentration).

The traditional yogic path to a meditative state is concentration, or focusing your awareness on a single point: a mantra, a candle flame, a visual image, etc. Another path toward meditation is mindfulness, simply attending to all thoughts, emotions, and sensations that arise as you sit. Both routes to meditation can effectively decrease stress and allow you to discover discover the stillness and peace inside you. The following technique melds the benefits of both concentration and mindfulness. You may want to record yourself reading the instructions, leaving the necessary gaps of time for silence.

## BASIC TECHNIQUE

1. Find a place where you won't be disturbed for 30 minutes. Sit in a Simple Sitting Pose (*Sukhasana*)—legs crossed, spine tall, and eyes closed.

2. Practice one, two, or all three of the Breathing Exercises (*Pranayama*) described on pages 104–107. This should take about 3–5 minutes altogether.

3. With your eyes still closed, observe your breath. Notice what happens during a breath: what part of your body moves on an inhalation, on an exhalation? What does your breath sound like? Is your breath shallow? Deep? Somewhere in between? Just observe without changing anything about your breath.

4. Now choose an aspect of your breath to focus on. Choose something lively that you can keep your attention fixed on: perhaps the sound of your breath or the sensation of your rib cage rising

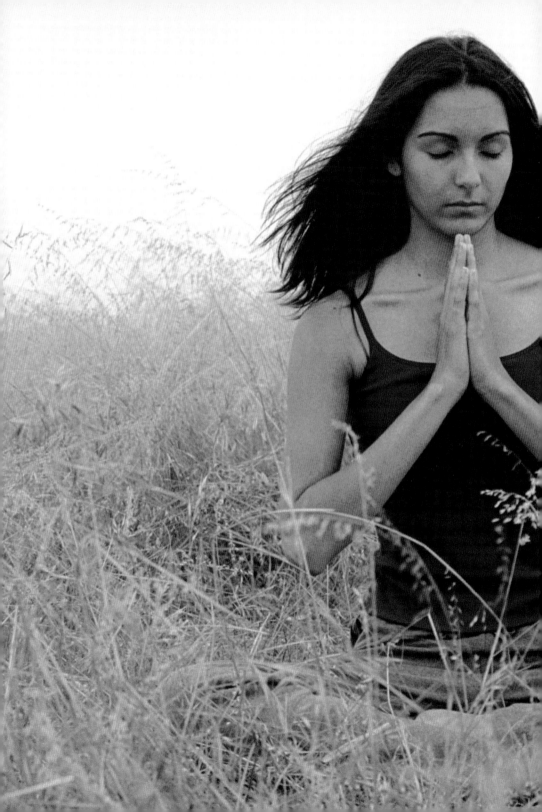

and falling. Spend the next 5 to 20 minutes attending to your breath. (Start with 5, work up to 20.)

- If a thought occurs, make a note of it. You can even identify it as "memory" or "fantasy," and then let it pass by without getting involved in it.
- If a physical sensation occurs, make a note of it. Label it as "tingling in feet . . . cold hands . . . pressure in knee . . ." and then let it go.
- If an emotion emerges, make a note of it. Identify it as "anger" or "sadness," etc.
- If a noise happens in the background, make a note of it and let it go.
- Don't focus on disruptions—accept all the thoughts, all the feelings, all the noises without judgment, and then bring your awareness back to your breath.

5. After your allotted time, keep your eyes closed for another minute or two. Just rest.

6. Slowly open your eyes. Take a few deep breaths, or perhaps a rousing round of Rapid Diaphragmatic Breathing (*Kapalabhati*; see page 106).

7. If you had any interesting insights or ideas during your meditation, write them down. Otherwise, let the experience go and get back to your life.

### *Modifications*
- If being in Simple Sitting Pose (*Sukhasana*) for 20 minutes doesn't feel right for your hips or knees, sit in a chair, on a bed,

or against a wall. Your comfort is more important than your ability to stay stock-still. But do stay upright to avoid dozing.

- Instead of watching your breath, you may substitute a mantra (a sound or word). Some examples are "peace" or "OM" or "shalom." Watch how the meaning of your word changes and how the sound and pronunciation mutate continuously. If you want to learn more about mantra meditation, find a qualified teacher to give you a mantra.

- Focusing *too* hard on your breath or on a sound can work against the process. Keep your focus light and flexible. If you feel your jaw clenching or a headache coming on, know that you might be trying too hard. Remind yourself, "It's easy."

- If thoughts or emotions rise up that are mildly irritating or disturbing, see if you can simply observe the sensations that those thoughts induce. Observe your irritation as if it were a passing cloud.

- If thoughts or emotions come up that frighten or upset you, take a deep breath, rest for a moment, and slowly open your eyes. You don't need to force yourself into confronting painful feelings. You might want to go do something very physical—a round of Sun Salutation (*Surya Namaskar*) or a brisk walk up and down some stairs—to get yourself back into your normal state of consciousness and try meditating again later.

- If you find yourself dozing off, try sitting in a *slightly* less comfortable position. If that doesn't work, get up and do a few vigorous rounds of Sun Salutation (*Surya Namaskar*) or some jumping jacks, and then sit again. Figure out if your dozing is a way to escape facing your thoughts and feelings, or if it is a genuine cry for more sleep.

We always meditate. We haven't missed a day in 28 years! And we do our best to do our system of breath/movement work every day. We often do a modified version of it in airports and on airplanes. When meditating on planes, we just don't mind the outside noise. Now we have something new we're using: noise-canceling earphones that block out a lot of the roar.

—Kathlyn Hendricks, Ph.D., and Gay Hendricks, Ph.D., authors of *Conscious Loving: The Journey to Co-Commitment* (Bantam Books)

### *Benefits*

- Increases mental clarity.
- Reduces blood pressure.
- Boosts levels of endorphins and other opoid (opium like) neuropeptides in the brain cells.
- Increases concentration and focus.
- Deepens awareness of the world.
- Gives you the opportunity to see the contents of your mind and to understand that you are not your thoughts.
- Allows you to approach a state of union with your higher self, which is the chief aim of yoga.

## MEDITATING ON THE ROAD

Once you begin a meditation program, you'll want to take it on the road with you. The question is how to fit it in while you're traveling? Some people, such as the Dalai Lama, have no trouble practicing on planes, trains, and in noisy public spaces. If this works for you, use your time in transit to go within. Bring foam earplugs to block out noise. Remember that airport meditation rooms (formerly known as "chapels") are a common sight in the U.S. and abroad.

If you've tried this route and it just doesn't work for you, you may need to be flexible about how you get your mind-work in. Its benefits depend on doing it regularly, especially if you are using a mantra. The sound vibration of a mantra establishes itself as neural pattern, but this pattern remains vivid only if it's repeated regularly. So if you truly believe that you don't have 20 minutes in the morning and 20 minutes in the afternoon to sit for your mantra repetition or mindfulness practice, then try 5 minutes. Better 5 minutes twice a day than an hour once every 3 or 4 days.

Another way you can include your meditation practice into your travel is to incorporate it into whatever activities you have planned. An example of this would be to transform a trip to the museum into an exploration of mindfulness. Find a gallery in the museum that isn't too crowded. Sit for a moment on a bench, if there's one available, and center yourself. Then devote more time than you normally would to drinking in each work of art. If you typically spend a minute gazing at a painting, commit to spending 5 minutes to really looking. Breathe steadily. Observe the painting strictly in terms of colors, then shapes, then textures. Observe the framing. Observe your response to the painting. Be open and accepting of any disruptions to your focus, and then gently bring your focus back to the painting.

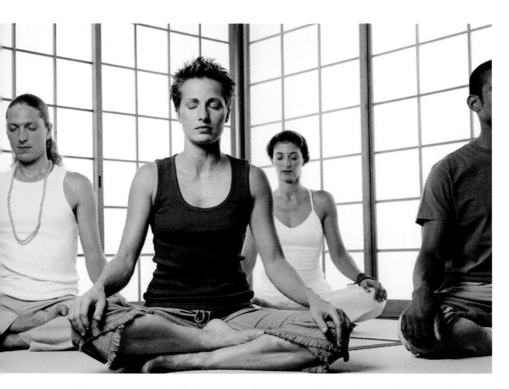

You can apply this same focus to things less pleasant than a painting. If you're traveling on business and are convinced that you don't have time to meditate, try taking one mindless task from your work and turning it into a mindful task. Bring every scrap of your attention to the details. Breathe steadily. You may find that the formerly unpalatable or dull job has become a little deeper.

## GUIDED MEDITATIONS

While not meant to take the place of a regular meditation practice, guided meditations are effective tools for self-discovery, stress management, and spiritual growth. They have specific themes, such as for peace and safety or for love, or they are intended to be done at specific times of the day, such as morning or evening. When done in partnership with a travel companion (one person reads the meditation while the other listens), these guided meditations can also be a powerful bonding experience.

## HOW TO USE THE GUIDED MEDITATIONS

The guided meditations in this book can be done in different ways. If you are traveling alone, you can record the meditations on a cassette before your trip, making sure you pause for the amount of time indicated, and then play the meditations on a portable cassette player. Or you can simply read the meditation to yourself (either aloud or silently) a few times so that its essence stays with you. Then close your eyes and begin the process, recalling each step. If you are traveling with a companion, or your family, you can each take turns being the reader/leader and the listener/follower.

Once you are in the meditation, see if you can keep your mind focused on the instructions without straining. When you notice your attention wandering, acknowledge whatever has captured your attention (whether it's a physical sensation, thought, or sound in the room) and then gently return your attention to the meditation instructions.

All of these meditations are brief enough to fit into your travel schedule. If you find you want more out of your session, feel free to repeat the script.

## HOW TO START A SESSION

Find a time and place that allows for maximum privacy and comfort and minimum distractions. Just like an *asana* session, a guided meditation session can be enhanced by the use of incense, candles, and gentle music, but none of these things is necessary.

Begin each guided meditation session with the deep relaxation technique Yogic Sleep (see pages 100–104). If you don't have time for the full deep relaxation process, simply sit comfortably, or lie down, and allow your entire body to let go. Take a few deep, slow breaths and then begin the meditation.

## HOW TO END A SESSION

Bring your awareness back to your breathing and take a few full, slow breaths. Allow your body to move freely. Sit comfortably for a few minutes before you get up and resume your activity. Drinking a glass of fresh, clean water provides a nice transition.

## FOR THE MORNING

This meditation prepares you for your busy day ahead.

- Breathe in and out, slowly and deeply, feeling the refreshing morning air. (Pause for 30 seconds.)

- As you inhale, breathe in energy and confidence. (Pause for 30 seconds.)

- As you exhale, release tension and fatigue. (Pause for 30 seconds.)

- Again, breathe in energy and confidence. (Pause for 30 seconds.)

- And exhale tension and fatigue. (Pause for 30 seconds.)

- Today's a new day, a chance to start again. (Pause for 30 seconds.)

- Feel yourself releasing the past, releasing yesterday. (Pause for 30 seconds.)

- Visualize the activities of your day ahead. (Pause for 30 seconds.)

- See yourself joyfully completing all your tasks.
  (Pause for 30 seconds.)

- See all your interactions with people as harmonious. You are pure
  peace, interacting with pure peace. (Pause for 30 seconds.)

- During the day, you will remember yourself as pure peace.
  (Pause for 30 seconds.)

- Bring your awareness back to your breath. (Pause for 30 seconds.)

- Allow your body to move freely and start your new day.
  (Pause for 30 seconds.)

## FOR THE EVENING

This meditation is best done in bed before you sleep. If you are using a tape recorder, make sure the sound of the tape turning off isn't jarring—and remember to put out any candles before drifting off.

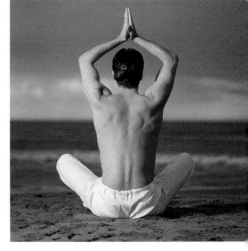

- Breathe in and out, slowly and
  deeply, feeling the calm night air
  and the comfort and safety of bed.
  (Pause for 30 seconds.)

- As you inhale, breathe in peace and
  relaxation. (Pause for 30 seconds.)

- As you exhale, release tension and worry. (Pause for 30 seconds.)

- Again, breathe in peace and relaxation. (Pause for 30 seconds.)

- And exhale tension and worry. (Pause for 30 seconds.)

- Let go of whatever happened today. (Pause for 30 seconds.)

- Feel yourself releasing the events of the day. (Pause for 30 seconds.)

- See yourself blissfully falling into a deep, refreshing sleep. (Pause for 30 seconds.)

- Bring your awareness back to your breath. (Pause for 30 seconds.)

- Continue to observe your breath as you slip into a peaceful sleep.

This meditation helps to soothe your mind when worries and anxieties take over.

- Take a few moments to watch your breath. Notice how effortless your breath is. (Pause for a minute.)

- Notice the thoughts in your mind. See how effortless the thoughts are. You are not your thoughts . . . . You are the witness to your thoughts. (Pause for a minute.)

- Knowing that you are not your body and not your thoughts, go

You have to ask yourself when you travel, "What is the cost of not practicing?" You can look at *asana* practice as something that you inflict on yourself, or you can look at it is as an expression, a celebration. You'll learn a lot either way, and it can lead you to a broader definition of "practice"—not just what happens on the mat, but how you approach other people and how you treat yourself.

When I'm on the road, a timer is God's gift to the universe. It helps make time for meditation. Your mind may throw up barriers saying, "I don't have time to meditate." But the timer says, "Yes you do, you have 10 minutes!"

—Judith Lasater, Ph.D., P.T., teacher, physical therapist, author of *Relax and Renew: Restful Yoga for Stressful Times* and *Living Your Yoga: Finding the Spiritual in Everyday Life* (Rodmell Press)

deeper and feel the peace at the core of your being. (Pause for 30 seconds.)

- Peace inside you. (Pause for 30 seconds.)

- Peace surrounding you. (Pause for 30 seconds.)

- In the center of your being there is only peace. (Pause for 30 seconds.)

- You are perfectly safe. (Pause for 30 seconds.)

- Safety inside you. (Pause for 30 seconds.)

- Safety surrounds you. (Pause for 30 seconds.)

- Imagine this peace and safety as a soft glowing light. See the light surrounding your body. (Pause for 30 seconds.)

- Imagine the light extending out in all directions. Peace and safety above. Peace and safety below. Peace and safety behind. Peace and safety in front of you, guiding you through the day, smoothing the way ahead. (Pause 30 seconds.)

- Know that you're safe and at peace at all times. You can bring forth the peace and safety at the center of your being at all times. (Pause for 30 seconds.)

- Bring the awareness back to your breath. (Pause for 30 seconds.)

- Allow your body to move freely. (Pause for 30 seconds.)

## FOR LOVE

This meditation is based on the traditional Buddhist Lovingkindness, or *Metta*, meditation. This feels great, especially if you are traveling by yourself and feeling lonely, or if your traveling party includes people with whom you have a difficult relationship.

- Feel yourself sinking into the present moment. (Pause for 30 seconds.)

- Contact your heart center. Visualize it as a glowing light in the middle of your chest, emanating warmth. (Pause for 10 seconds.)

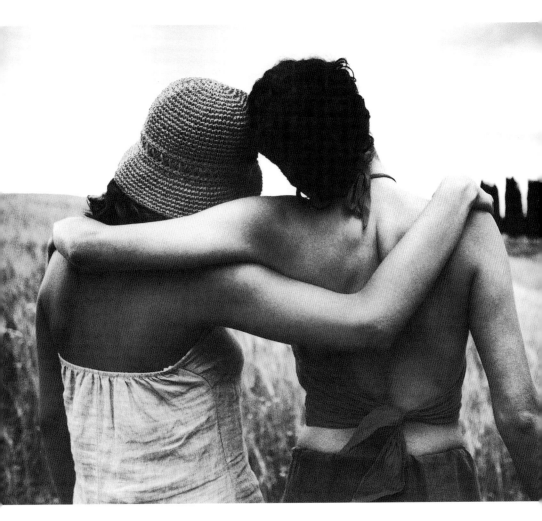

• Imagine a person you love deeply. Feel the love in your heart for this person. Imagine that this love glows through your entire being. (Pause for 10 seconds.)

• Feel that glowing love fill the room. (Pause for 10 seconds.)

• Feel that love radiate out into the world, reaching that person, and all other sentient beings. (Pause for 30 seconds.)

- Now visualize a person you feel neutral towards: a stranger, a celebrity, or a co-worker. (Pause for 10 seconds.)

- Again, contact your heart center. Feel that glowing love and compassion in your heart for this person. Imagine your love wrapping around this person and filling them with peace. (Pause for 30 seconds.)

- Now visualize a person you are having difficulty with. (Pause for 10 seconds.)

- Send this person all the love, compassion, and goodwill that illuminates your heart. (Pause for 30 seconds.)

- See this person succeeding in all he or she wants to do. See this person receiving all the love he or she needs. (Pause for 30 seconds.)

- Now visualize yourself. Send yourself all the love, compassion, and goodwill that illuminates your heart. (Pause for 30 seconds.)

- See yourself succeeding in all you want to do. See yourself receiving all the love you need. (Pause for 30 seconds.)

- Say to yourself, mentally or aloud, "May all beings be happy. May all beings have peace. May all beings be free."

- Bring your awareness back to your breath. (Pause for 10 seconds.)

- Allow your body to move freely.

## FOR HEALING

If you are feeling under the weather, this meditation will put you in contact with your innate healing potential. For best results, set aside enough time to experience a complete Yogic Sleep (see pages 100–104) deep-relaxation session prior to this guided meditation. Once you are deeply relaxed, begin.

• Imagine you are surrounded by a brilliant white light. See it glowing all around you. (Pause for 10 seconds.)

• This light is the innate power of your body/mind to heal itself. (Pause for 10 seconds.)

• As the light surrounds you, acknowledge the miracle of your body, the way it functions so efficiently and supports your soul. Honor the magnificence of your perfect body. (Pause for 10 seconds.)

• If there is tension or dysfunction somewhere in your body, allow the light to center on that part of your body. Know that any temporary disturbances can be calmed and healed by the flow of light. (Pause for 30 seconds.)

• Feel the light gently dissolve any blockages of energy, allowing the healing energy to restore you to wholeness. (Pause for 30 seconds.)

• If there is pain or discomfort in your body, allow yourself to feel the sensations of pain without resistance. Find where the pain starts, where it travels to, and how it changes. (Pause for 30 seconds.)

- Now visualize the light surrounding the source of pain. Feel the light healing and soothing you. (Pause for 30 seconds.)

- Imagine your body functioning in complete wholeness and perfection. Remember a time when you felt completely alive and joyful and healthy. If nothing comes to mind, simply imagine what it would feel like, what it would look like, and what it would be like to be completely healed. (Pause for a minute.)

- Now let that image go and affirm that all is well. (Pause for 10 seconds.)

- Bring your awareness back to your breath. (Pause for 30 seconds.)

- Allow your body to move freely.

## WALKING MEDITATION

This meditation helps bring peace and awareness to every step of your journey.

- Begin by standing. (Pause for 10 seconds.)

- Become aware of your feet touching the earth. Relax your feet. (Pause for 10 seconds.)

- Become aware of the sensations in your body. (Pause for 10 seconds.)

- Begin to walk slowly at an easy pace. (Pause for 10 seconds.)

- Focus on the sensation of your feet contacting the ground.
  (Pause for 10 seconds.)

- Notice your heel hitting the ground first, then the slow roll of your
  foot, and then your toes bending and lifting your foot off the
  ground. (Pause for 10 seconds.)

- Continue noticing the sensations and activity of your feet.
  (Pause for 30 seconds.)

- Become aware of the sensations and activity of your calves and
  shins. (Pause for 30 seconds.)

- Become aware of the sensations and activity of your knees.
  (Pause for 30 seconds.)

- Become aware of the sensations and activity of your thighs and
  quadriceps. (Pause for 30 seconds.)

- Become aware of the sensations and activity of your hips and
  pelvis. (Pause for 30 seconds.)

- Become aware of the sensations and activity of your arms and
  shoulders. (Pause for 30 seconds.)

- Become aware of the sensations and activity of your neck, head,
  and face. (Pause for 30 seconds.)

- Become aware of the totality of your physical experience.
  (Pause for 30 seconds.)

- Become aware of the relationship between you and your environment. (Pause for 30 seconds.)

- Now bring your focus back inside and become aware once again of the sensation of your feet. (Pause for 30 seconds.)

- Notice your heel hitting the ground first, then the slow roll of your foot, and then your toes bending and lifting your foot off the ground. (Pause for 10 seconds.)

- Continue noticing the sensations and activity of your feet. (Pause for 30 seconds.)

- Turn off the tape recorder for as long as you want to continue your walking meditation. When you are ready to wind down, turn the tape recorder back on.

- Now stop walking. (Pause for 30 seconds.)

- Become aware of your feet touching the earth. (Pause for 10 seconds.)

- Notice if you feel any more focused, relaxed, or in harmony with your surroundings. If not, let the experience go. If so, see if you can retain a bit of this groundedness for the rest of your day.

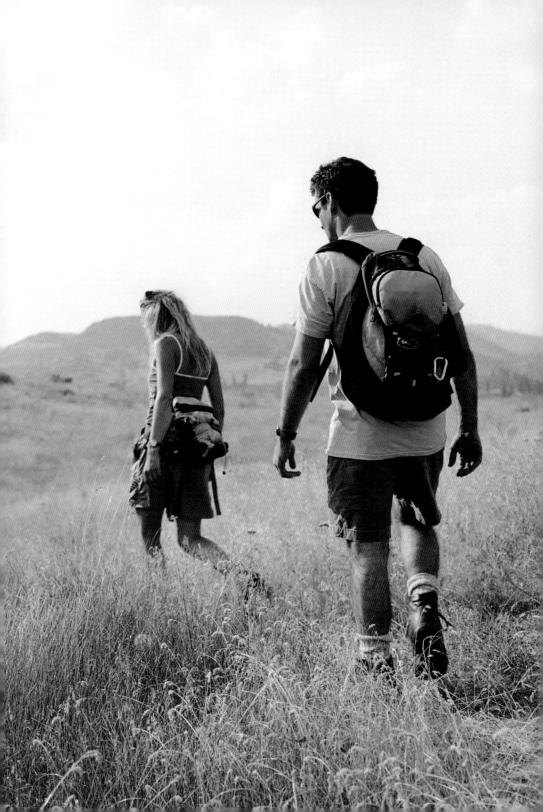

# INDEX

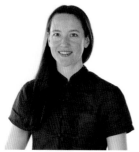

## ABOUT THE AUTHOR
PAULA CARINO has been practicing hatha yoga and meditation for over 10 years, and has been a certified instructor since 1999. She teaches at Integral Yoga Institute in New York City and has also taught at a variety of yoga studios, fitness centers, and corporations in and around New York. She is a songwriter and musician who performs regularly with her band. A New Jersey native, she currently lives in Brooklyn with her husband and two hounds. She actually loves airplane travel and wrote most of this book in the air.

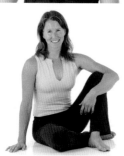

## ABOUT THE MODEL
ZELINA BLAGDEN is a yoga instructor and practitioner who received her training through Alison West and David Swensen. She has taught yoga in California and New Mexico. She currently lives and teaches privately in New York City.